£1.50

MENTAL HANDICAP NURSING AND CARE

HUMAN HORIZONS SERIES

MENTAL HANDICAP NURSING AND CARE

by

Victoria Shennan

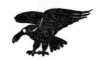

A CONDOR BOOK
SOUVENIR PRESS (E & A) LTD

Acknowledgements
Thanks are due to my husband, Dr Edward T. Shennan, to my children and grandchildren, to the many students I have been privileged to teach, to past and present colleagues, especially those of the National Society for Mentally Handicapped Children, and to my friends who are mentally handicapped, particularly Joseph John Deacon, fellow author, and his team at St Lawrence's Hospital, Caterham, from all of whom I have learned more than I can ever hope to teach.

Photographs
All illustrations are copyright to the National Society for Mentally Handicapped Children.

First published 1980 by Souvenir Press (Educational & Academic) Ltd,
43 Great Russell Street, London WC1B 3PA
and simultaneously in Canada

ISBN 0 285 64903 5 casebound
ISBN 0 285 64902 7 paperback

Printed in Great Britain by
Clarke, Doble & Brendon Ltd,
Plymouth and London

Contents

6 CONTENTS

Appendix

Foreword

It may seem to most of us that the world of the mentally retarded person is a strange and mysterious one. We may feel that we must make great efforts to cross the frontier between 'us' and 'them', and we may never feel that we have penetrated very far.

Sometimes we may feel that the effort of understanding is too great, and the rewards of communication too few, to merit the demands that work with mentally handicapped people makes upon all in daily contact with them.

But suddenly, often quite unheralded, we make a break-through, which results, perhaps, in a communion of spirit, rather than a contact of minds. It is this experience which rewards the many parents and professional workers and gives them encouragement and hope.

We are all constantly learning more about ourselves and our world, and the possibilities for helping mentally handicapped people to achieve the dignity of their human condition. This is the ultimate aim of all who are involved in their care.

As more and more mentally handicapped people live among us, their special needs must not be forgotten, nor must they be denied skills which are available to us all.

This book is not concerned with the specialised skills of the registered mental nurse, nor with the psychiatric treatment available in hospitals.

It is concerned with the application of simple general nursing skills to the benefit of mentally handicapped people, aimed at maintaining health, rather than curing preventable disease, and with introducing to nurses and care staff some of the skills of other professions which can be used in the daily personal care of mentally handicapped people, to develop their abilities to the maximum of which they are capable.

To cover the whole field in one small handbook permits only

a brief introduction to each speciality, and to each aspect and stage of mentally handicapped people.

There are no 'correct' techniques—each person, parent, nurse or helper will discover his own methods of helping individuals which are not mentioned in any handbook.

To all who wish to work with mentally handicapped people, I recommend listening to handicapped children and adults, patiently and often, as they try to express their own needs; to observe closely those who cannot speak to discover what they think and feel; and to use imagination and enterprise to obtain for them the services they need, but cannot ask for for themselves.

Introduction

Students entering the caring professions for mental handicap will come from many disciplines and into an entirely new concept of care.

For many years, medical and nursing personnel were almost alone in providing for the life-time care of mentally handicapped people, but today, with the recognition that, in the majority of cases, mentally handicapped people do not need specifically medical and nursing care, but education, support and appropriate therapy, the role of the nurse and, more importantly, the institutional care of mentally handicapped people is under review.

In 1971 the Government issued a White Paper, *Better Services for the Mentally Handicapped* (Cmnd. 4683), which outlined plans for a change of policy for their care, and laid particular emphasis on questioning the routine admission to hospital of such people. It concluded that 'the aim should be to fix for each area as early a date as possible after which hospitals will not be asked to admit any more people who need residential, rather than hospital care'.

So, gradually, the very large number of people, over 50,000 in 1978, at present in hospitals of this special type—subnormality hospitals—will be reduced, though a greater proportion of those remaining will be ageing and aged. Instead, mentally handicapped people will live among us in the community.

The Committee of Enquiry into Mental Handicap Nursing and Care, under the chairmanship of Peggy Jay, reported its findings to Government in 1979, and stated, once again, that the old concept of hospital care, and nursing and medical supervision, needs urgent review.

But what is to replace it? A fresh consideration of the label 'hospital' and 'home'—a 'Home', or a 'home' is needed.

If we think that the word 'hospital' means a place where people go to be cured of disease, then it is the wrong word to use for a place where mentally handicapped people live at home; equally, many an establishment labelled 'a home', has little relationship to the home most of us know, the place which not only offers us protection from the outside world, a place where we can cast off our cares and worries and relax, but also gives us privacy, a chance to be ourselves and to enjoy individual pleasures.

So we must be ready for the very considerable changes which will take place in all the professions concerned with mental handicap, be ready to review our own concepts of our careers, our status and the present hierachies in this period of rapid change, but remembering also that the one fixed point is the handicapped child or adult in his small private world who looks to us for stability, continuity of care and compassion, and help in reaching his potential for living.

There are some certainties: primarily, that among this group of people living today, there will always be individuals in need of more support than the average member of society. By reason of their handicap they will not be able to meet the demands of the ever-increasing technological bias of our world.

They will need care, in the true and best sense of caring, by others who choose to spend their working lives in this vocation; and, be they called nurses, teachers, social workers, house-parents, or fulfill all these roles as natural parents, they will need all the expertise of each other to give the best help to the handicapped child or adult.

In this sense, the place where this help is given is not material. For some years yet the hospital will continue to be a home for adults who are not able to function in the outside world; and there will always be some children so grievously afflicted that they need to be within immediate reach of skilled medical and nursing attention. But wherever this may be, it will always be primarily their home, so those who work there have the added duty, over and above the medical and educational care they provide, to concern themselves with the quality of life children and adults enjoy.

An insight into the shape of things to come can be seen in the present educational provisions for mentally handicapped young

children. For many years, no support, no help at all was available
in the vulnerable first years of life, and families struggled as best
they could with the care and education of the infant. Now, from
the earliest months, and even before the age of two years, educational facilities are available to handicapped babies in most areas.
Physiotherapy advice enables the parents to handle the child in
the best way and helps to prevent lifelong physical disability.
Other ancillary services, though by no means adequate, begin to
be called upon.

One Local Authority, writing about its personal services to the
mentally handicapped says;

> 'Our 120-place ESN(S) School will also have attached to it a
> 32-place hospital for children attending the School, of a kind
> who are at present catered for in a hospital. This new linked
> hospital will be controlled by the Area Health Authority.
> Although a hospital in name, it is in essence a unit of four
> separate homes each making provision for eight children in
> the age ranges of 2–19.'

A hospital of eight beds?—labelled so, for administrative con-
venience, but hardly what most people would envisage as a
hospital.

It is possible that the present subnormality hospitals will become
resource centres, where staff with particular skills are based whilst
working in the community; that they may provide specialist
facilities for speech training, for physiotherapy and remedial
gymnastics and other services which mentally handicapped people
need in greater proportion than the rest of the community. But
equally, if mentally handicapped people are to live lives as nearly
like ours as possible, they will sometimes be ill and need medical
and nursing care, sometimes need counselling, sometimes need
legal advice, sometimes need financial help. Those who provide
these services will need to understand the condition of mental
handicap, how it affects those who suffer under it, how present
attitudes and provisions have evolved, and the direction that
future care will take.

Students commencing a career in the nursing and care of mentally handicapped people can take heart from the acknowledgement of their role by Professor Peter Mittler,* Chairman of the National Development Group for the Mentally Handicapped, in his 1978 Report to the Secretary of State, that they are 'the backbone of the mental handicap service'.

The quality of the backbone is its great strength, its ability to bear the heaviest physical burdens; and its supreme flexibility. It is also the nerve channel which activates all the other vital body functions—not perhaps a bad description of the role of the caring personnel in the field of mental handicap.

*Helping Mentally Handicapped People in Hospital. Department of Health and Social Security. October 1978. Chapter 7, para. 2.8.

SECTION ONE

A General View

A General View

For centuries past, those among us who were handicapped by a reduced capacity to understand the demands of their environment and of the society in which they lived, were compelled to endure whatever quality of life might be deemed by the rest of society appropriate to their needs.

At best, this life style tended to be custodial, and attempted to replace the individual's inability to make major decisions about his own daily life a regular daily programme, interpreted by a variety of attendants : sometimes doctors or nurses, sometimes care assistants, sometimes the parent of the person involved. At worst it became a life of virtual imprisonment for the handicapped person, with no aspect of his life at his own disposal, and no recognition of his rights as a person.

It is only very recently that the needs of mentally handicapped persons have begun to be considered on the same level as those of other handicapped people—the blind, the deaf, the physically handicapped and the very young and very aged—as being special to their condition, but no justification for excluding them from rights enjoyed by other citizens.

Similarly, the recognition that physically handicapped people may have little else in common than their handicap, is at last being applied to the mentally handicapped as well.

WHAT IS MENTAL HANDICAP?

Mental handicap is a condition which makes life a lot more difficult for those who are affected and it is a condition which is a life-long disability, and, at this time, has no medical cure, but is capable of amelioration by appropriate education and care.

If a person is born without a fully functioning limb, as was the case with many of the thalidomide children, it is a condition which cannot be cured. What can be done, and is daily more excitingly seen to be done, is to replace the lost abilities by man-made imitation of the lost part, and to stimulate the abilities which remain to minimise the handicap of the missing limb.

Those who have the misfortune to be born without, or to lose during their life, some of the functions of the brain, can be helped by full stimulation of the abilities remaining. The science of neuro-surgery, for example, is one branch of medicine in which the frontiers of knowledge are increasing daily. We know something of how the brain functions, which areas are responsible for speech and communication, which for memory, which for imagination, and so on, but each advance tells us even more of how little we really know.

What we *do* know, is that if some part of the brain is damaged, or is not developed by the time of birth, certain functions will never be adequately performed.

But just as a blind man develops extra sensitivity in other areas —for example, in the sense of touch—we are increasingly aware that deficiencies in some areas of the brain are compensated for by others, and that by concentrating upon the development and full potential of the areas which are undamaged, much of the handicap can be reduced.

We also know that such remedial teaching and stimulation must begin as early as possible to achieve the maximum result and that, sadly, mentally handicapped adults who are given education only later in life, have less chance to achieve the full potential of their other abilities than young children. But equally, we know also that there is no age at which an individual is totally incapable of new learning.

So, mental handicap is a condition which is not capable of cure, but is capable of improvement by concentration upon what can be done, rather than on what cannot.

INITIAL ATTITUDES

Most people tend to withdraw from anyone who is 'different'— 'not like the rest of us'—'not normal', and you may experience this inital reaction yourself when you first see a person who is handicapped, either physically or mentally. You may also feel that this rejection is unworthy, and should be hidden.

It may help if you know that it is unconscious and instinctive, and not something which should be denied or pushed away without explanation.

In every species there is an in-built mechanism to reproduce only the standard model—only the individual most closely resembling the 'normal' specimen. This is because, by the process of evolution over many centuries, each species has evolved the individual best able to survive and reproduce. All other, less perfect specimens, perish. The white blackbird will be destroyed by other birds, the wild animal born blind will not survive.

Only man, with his superior abilities, can make use of the non-typical specimen. From the non-typical man, the species is enriched by painters, poets and mystics, and mankind learns and grows by the toleration within the human family of many who are less able to care for themselves, or to contribute to society on a purely basic level.

For those of us who are entrusted with the role of helpers and friends to the less able, there is a particular need to understand those who are mentally handicapped, and to understand fully what their difficulties are.

INTELLIGENCE

To most people, the quality of intelligence is something which can be measured by means of tests, can be analysed to give a prediction of the capacity of the mind, and can often be considered to give some judgement of the value of the individual to the rest of society.

Intelligence is often spoken of as if is were an accurate and unchanging factor of the human personality, like the temperature of the human body.

But though it is fair to say that most human beings have a normal temperature ranging from 97°F to 99°F, it is by no means an accurate scientific statement. Variations in normal temperature can be caused by the time of day when it is recorded, by the environment or clothing of the individual, by transpiration of fluid, and, of course, by the local temperature of the mouth if that is where the temperature is recorded. If the mean of 100 is taken as the measure of intelligence, this measure is obtained by a standardised test, which, though reasonably accurate under normal conditions, is subject to just as many variables as the temperature in making an assessment of the individual.

So we can take the measure of intelligence in a mentally handicapped person as a rough basic guide, not as a fixed reading which will never vary.

Intelligence test results have been used as a guide for administrative procedures, so it is necessary for us to know what they mean.

If 100 is taken as the measure of average intelligence, we can expect persons with a level of 70–100 to function just like everyone else in the community. When the measured levels of intelligence drop markedly below the 70 level, however, the performance of the person, measured against the 'normal' level of 100, will be materially affected. When that levels drops to 50 it will be very noticeable that the person is functioning well below average levels. It is generally accepted that just under 2 per cent of the whole population have I.Q. levels below 70, and that 2 or 3 persons in every 1,000 will be mentally handicapped to some degree.

In the absence of a more accurate measure, the intelligence test gives a quick rule of thumb method of classifying the ability of a person; for want of any better single test, it is used, like the body temperature level, to decide if further assessment is needed.

So that we all know what is meant by mental handicap, and to give a rough idea of the various levels of handicap, there have been many classifications based upon the intelligence quotients (I.Q.). These classifications have varied over the years from one country an another, but the WHO has suggested that most countries would agree upon the following formula, as stated in the International Classification of Diseases (1965).

Grades of retardation

Borderline	I.Q.	68%–85%
Mild	I.Q.	52%–67%
Moderate	I.Q.	36%–51%
Severe	I.Q.	20%–35%
Profound	I.Q.	below 20%

In Britain, the term 'mentally handicapped' has been offically adopted, and the Mental Health Act of 1959 defines mental handicap as affecting 'persons who are incapable of leading an independent life, or of guarding against serious exploitation when of an age to do so' (Section V, para. 2). Persons previously described in law as idiots, imbeciles or feeble-minded, generally speaking, had measured I.Q. levels of less than 50, and were classified *'severely subnormal'*. The Mental Health Act of 1959 also identified a group of people who were classified as *'subnormal*—a condition which was susceptible to medical treatment or special care or training', with I.Q. levels above 50. The I.Q. level of 50 was crucial for admission to Special Education. Those below it were deemed *'ineducable'*.

No such educational distinction now exists. Every child is deemed capable of some education, appropriate to his need and ability and modern concepts suggest that there is greater hope for special education and training for people with I.Q. levels below 50 if they receive individual programmes early in life.

The Mental Health Act of 1959 is now under review and many concepts relating to mental handicap will be changed. There is a considerable body of opinion which demands that mental handicap be removed from the Act entirely, and that mental illness only be covered by the new Act.

LEGAL ASPECTS

Mentally handicapped people have rights in common law, just as everyone else, and have duties in common law unless they have been declared incompetent to be responsible for their actions.

It is reasonable to assume that those in daily contact with and caring for mentally handicapped people of all levels of ability will know what each person can be expected to understand. It is, then, the duty of the helper to instruct the handicapped person clearly in such areas of daily life where he may be in conflict with the law, and, where his understanding is insufficient for him to profit by instruction, to take such steps as are needed to protect him.

For example, no one expects a small child to understand that he should not urinate in the street, unless he is told, and unless he is old enough to understand what he is told. A child of five years is hardly likely to be summonsed for causing a public nuisance by so doing.

An adult can be prosecuted for such an offence, therefore those in charge of adults who are not capable of understanding that it is an offence are *themselves* liable in the event of an offence.

It follows that nurses and care staff who have to instruct groups of people in generally acceptable conduct will decide how far each person can understand, and how much the responsibility for his conduct devolves upon the helper.

In a professional situation, helpers are protected by the employing authority against professional mistakes, provided they have acted within the code of conduct laid down in their employment.

It is impossible to lay down exact rules to cover every situation, but helpers in an institution should always ask advice if they have doubts about any handicapped person's ability to go out alone, for instance, or to use knives or cookers, or to bath alone. If it is felt that a person is progressing and could be given more freedoms which involve a degree of risk, the first thing to do is to consult with other team members.

Both the safety of the person and the safety of society must always be considered when a legal risk is involved, but the guiding principle is always, 'where is the responsibility?—can he carry this if I ensure his training is efficient, or must I?' This question must be asked and answered in all situations, not only in hospitals, but in Training Centres, hostels and in residential situations requiring supervision.

The legal position of mentally handicapped people in hospitals is defined under the Mental Health Act of 1959. Such people, both adults and children, may be admitted to hospital by their own wish, or that of their parents, as *informal* patients. These people are free to leave when they wish.

The Act also provided under certain circumstances for both mentally handicapped and medically ill people to be compulsorily detained in hospitals for treatment for their disability and/or for the protection of others. These people are not free to leave unless formally discharged by the psychiatrist in charge, or by a Court of Law.

Proposed changes

The Act is currently under review and there are some changes which may have far-reaching effects. It is proposed that a mentally handicapped person will in future be admitted to hospital *only* if he is unable to maintain himself in the community, with available community care, or if his condition has a prospect of benefit from treatment.

Certain nominated persons may however still have statutory powers to remove a mentally handicapped person into a place of safety or to keep him there for a limited period whilst proper consultation takes place.

The police may take such action, and there will be a time limit during which they may legally detain a person, 72 hours is suggested

A registered mental nurse may be given statutory power to detain a person in hospital or other place of safety for a short period—6 hours is suggested—so that a consultant may advise.

There would be only two grounds for admitting people to institutional care; that the admission is in the interest of health and safety of the person, or that it will protect others from harm.

Statutory powers mean that a person acting under these enactments is fully protected by law, and it is proposed that one further category of person 'an approved social worker' will also be given these duties.

Nurses and care assistants generally will not have these statutory powers, or protection. They may themselves need protection from a charge that they did not carry out duties, or behaved unreasonably in their contacts with mentally handicapped people, and some professional bodies provide legal protection cover to their members in return for fees for membership.

SECTION TWO

Diagnosis, Patterns of Care, Attitudes

How is Mental Handicap discovered?

Conditions diagnosed at birth

Conditions arising after birth

Prevalence and Incidence

Classification

Mildly and moderately retarded

Severely retarded

Profoundly retarded

Patterns of Care

Where are mentally handicapped people today?

Attitudes

Personal

Public

Parental

Professional

Causation

Genetic factors

Chromosomal factors

Infections

Birth Injuries

Environmental factors

Prematurity

Research

Diagnosis, Patterns of Care, Attitudes

HOW IS MENTAL HANDICAP DISCOVERED?

Very often, if the mentally handicapped child is the first child in the family, his handicap will not be finally diagnosed before his second year.

The grandparents or other relatives may say that the baby is 'slow', or the mother may feel that the baby is not quite like other babies, but it may take a long time for these fears to become concrete enough to lead them to seek expert diagnosis. Sometimes, the experts themselves are slow to recognise a handicap. On the other hand, some types of mental handicap are obvious at birth and the medical staff present will have to inform the parents that their child will need special care. The first information is crucial, and needs to be handled with great sensitivity : many bad mistakes have been made in the past in what the parents were told, and in the way they were told. It is easy to criticise, with hindsight, but we now know that so much depends upon the care and attention the infant receives from his earliest days that it is imperative that parents are told about mental handicap as soon, and as kindly, as possible. They will need time to absorb the initial shock, and to grieve for the healthy baby they have lost. Then they need to be given the vital information about what they can do for the child.

Conditions diagnosed at birth

Mongolism is usually immediately apparent, as is microcephaly, and other specific syndromes. More information will be given later on the various types of mental handicap, but the 'label' is on the *condition*, not on the child. In many cases the *condition* cannot be changed, and it is even more important to concentrate on the child, and begin at once to give the help he needs.

Birth injuries may result in damage to the brain, though the degree of damage and the resulting effects may not be immediately apparent.

The diagnosis of mental handicap is made in very much the same way as other medical diagnoses, by comparison with the normal. You will perhaps have seen that when an injury is sustained—a sprain or suspected fracture—that the doctor will compare the injured joint with the other normal one in case of doubt.

The measure of mental handicap is arrived at in a similar way. We know what normal babies can do at birth, then at various weeks of age before their second birthday. By careful obversation and testing we can see that these stages, sometimes called 'milestones of development', are reached in their proper order.

The healthy infant is born with the mental capacity to survive. He can adjust to his environment, and profit by experience. Very early he will turn his head to the side, if laid upon his face, to ensure that he can breathe freely; he will grip his mother's fingers or hair if he feels insecure; he will scream loudly if he is hungry or cold or in pain; and he will repeat this behaviour if he finds that it achieves the desired result.

We shall give more information on the simple developmental tests later, but it is enough to know that it is possible to tell very early in life, by watching for certain universal activities such as lifting the head and co-ordinating eye movements, that a child is mentally handicapped, and in what direction he will need most help.

Conditions arising after birth

There is a group of mentally handicapped people who were born healthy, but subsequently, through illness or accident, sustain damage to the brain resulting in mental handicap.

These conditions can be physical, caused by road accidents, infections or as the result of improper administration of drugs, vaccines or anaesthetics.

They can be developmental, resulting from abnormal experiences, such as having been locked away from others and isolated from human contact for long periods. Children who come as immigrants to a new society may appear to be retarded and those from very deprived social environments may underachieve to such an extent that they are classified mentally handicapped.

The need for experience in order to learn is fundamental to mankind, and there have been well documented cases of children socially and emotionally deprived who have suffered such damage that they are permanently mentally handicapped.

But in each and every case those who care for them, child or adult, must never accept that nothing can be done to improve the quality of their lives.

The human personality is capable of development in many and varied ways, and can be profoundly affected by the environment, by experience, and most of all, by the presence or absence of love.

PREVALENCE AND INCIDENCE

Confusion often arises between the *prevalence* of mentally handicapped people in a community and the *incidence* of the condition.

The incidence of mental handicap in any population is relatively stable : that is, that within certain limits, the same percentage of babies will be born with some degree of mental handicap everywhere in the world.

The incidence, like all other human conditions, may vary from time to time because of imposed changes—for example, from a new environmental factor such as pollution—but as in all such changes, the tendency is to revert to the norm. The fluctuations will not persist and the overall rate will remain constant. The theoretical proportion of mentally handicapped persons in the population has been studied by Professor Lionel Penrose, who suggested that given I.Q. 100 as normal, there would in any given population be born the same percentage of persons with less than average intelligence, as of persons with above average intelligence. In other words, there would be roughly the same number of mentally handicapped babies born as of exceptionally gifted ones.

Prevalence, on the other hand, means the number of persons *actually present* within the community who suffer from mental handicap, and it will readily be seen that this will depend upon many factors.

Given that mentally handicapped people are less able to defend themselves against the adverse factors in their daily living, it is obvious that in harsh conditions of excessive cold or heat, for example, or where there is inadequate food supply, the mentally handicapped infants will succumb first, thus leaving fewer in the community and a reduced prevalence.

In highly developed societies, there may well be a greater number of mentally handicapped people than the average, because the less harsh environmental conditions and greater care for the less fortunate citizens, enables them to survive. In the future, it may be that this balance will change as developments in preventive medicine discover potentially handicapped infants before birth, and terminations of such pregnancies increase.

Rural communities absorb into their societies many people of less than average intelligence, who are useful and contributing members of a society which relies upon basic skills of agriculture and husbandry. The technically advanced community can find fewer opportunities for the employment of mentally handicapped people.

CLASSIFICATION

The degree of mental handicap is useful only as a very rough guide to the ability of the person concerned and to the amount of help and guidance he will need in his daily life.

Mildly and moderately retarded people attend special schools for children called 'educationally subnormal' (ESN M), and many of these people will be able to take up employment in the community and live independent lives.

Severely retarded people (ESN S) receive education specially designed to develop the abilities they have, to counteract any disabling conditions imposed by their handicap, and to provide help appropriate to their adult lives.

Profoundly retarded people many receive only very basic contacts between their helpers and themselves, from childhood. They will always need a close degree of special care from others.

But it is very important to remember that each person is an individual and has all the rights of others. A profoundly handicapped person may not have profound physical disabilities— though he is often doubly handicapped in this way—and may have an easy amenable personality, whilst a mildly retarded person may have a severe physical handicap, such as a heart defect, or extreme emotional problems, perhaps due to difficult childhood conditions, which make for very great difficulties in his daily care.

So we need always to remember, when we meet a mentally handicapped child or adult for the first time, that what matters is the stage he is in *now* and what can be done to help and improve his life. What is past, what has caused or aggravated his state is done. We have to concentrate upon what we can do *now* to make his future more enjoyable and to discover those who can work with us to do so.

PATTERNS OF CARE

We have discovered that mental handicap occurs throughout the world and that provisions for the care and education of handicapped people vary accordingly to the country in which they live; but in each country there will probably be provision by the State (statutory provisions), as well as provision by other organisations.

Where no orderly form of national provision exists, the care of mentally handicapped people rests with their families and sometimes with charitable foundations and voluntary groups. Religious bodies, Christian and others, have often provided care for those who could not care for themselves, and continue to do so in many parts of the world.

There are caring individuals in all societies, who give such help either as a personal contribution, or by combining into groups with the declared aim of helping special sections of people with exceptional needs. Such groups often become politically active and force upon the government of the country an acceptance of the need to provide for the less able.

Statutory help will always be dependent upon public funds, and therefore upon public attitudes. This is why provision for the mentally handicapped varies so much in different countries.

In Britain we inherit our tradition of care from the industrial revolution of the nineteenth century.

From the mid eighteenth century, vast numbers of people left the small rural communities to live in huge urban conurbations, specifically for the purpose of work in the new factories. Whole families were uprooted, bringing with them into the cities their aged people, their sick and handicapped. Since the purpose of their move was to work, those who could not work presented a problem.

The problem had always existed, but in the smaller, rural community it could be contained. The village group could provide community care for the old, mutual support for widows and orphans, and some degree of care and occupation for people who were handicapped. Lower standards of hygiene and nutrition, and ignorance of the cause of many diseases, however, resulted in a high mortality rate among the less able, and, to some degree, was accepted as inevitable.

The tremendous changes imposed by urban living resulted in traumatic change for the families. Women working in factories could provide less care for children, who, in turn were quickly assimilated into the work force, sometimes as early as five years of age.

An awakening of national conscience, in Victorian times began to provide large institutions for the care of abandoned children, old people, and those physically ill. But the mentally handicapped and mentally ill presented a much greater problem. No-one knew how to treat the mentally ill, much less how to care for the mentally handicapped, or even how to distinguish between the two. But, increasingly humanitarian ideas would not tolerate any longer such barbaric institutions as Bedlam and other lunacy houses, where the mad were put on show for the entertainment of others.

New concepts demanded that special hospitals be built for both mentally ill and mentally handicapped. Because land was more easily available outside towns—where the factories swallowed up all available sites—they were often built in remote areas. They were very large institutions—the Victorians built and planned on a grand scale. These large subnormality hospitals with medical and professional nursing care (itself a new concept, dating only from Florence Nightingale's experience in the Crimean War of 1854–6) for the mentally handicapped, remain a legacy that Britain today would wish to lose. Other countries followed the British model—the old Commonwealth and some of the emerging industrial countries in Europe and America.

Countries such as Sweden and Denmark on the other hand, with smaller, more centralised organisation, have been able in this century to design national schemes and to implement them nationally, commencing with new ideas and new buildings from the start. Holland, too, used the re-building programmes of the postwar period, and war reparation funds, to expand and improve facilities for the mentally handicapped.

In some Federal countries—the United States, Canada and Australia for example—some of the provisions for the less able are undertaken by separate States, and therefore vary in quality from one area to the next.

Countries of the Third World, newly emerging from a rural economy, begin today where Victorian England began, but, with increased speed of communication and the international organisations such as WHO and UNESCO disseminating ideas, have in some ways a greater chance of providing imaginative community-based schemes for the mentally handicapped.

In Africa, some centres to serve villages have been set up in co-operation with urban hospitals. They take in for treatment and education, mentally ill and mentally handicapped people, with a member of the family or village to give daily care until the person can be returned to his community again. This scheme gives a two-fold benefit: the helper learns many techniques in his care of the original client; and he takes back to his village information and practical skills to assist in turn other similarly affected members.

This direct involvement of relatives and neighbours in a professional partnership in the care of mentally handicapped people is comparatively new in more developed countries. For a very long time, care was considered the prerogative of a hierachy of professionals, mainly medical, and parents were often told 'There is nothing you can do but have your child admitted to a subnormality hospital'. By implication, the parents were being advised to cut themselves off from the child; and indeed, many parents felt such a burden of guilt and grief that, in self-defence, they removed themselves permanently from contact with their child.

Others, often at great personal difficulty, visited hospitals many miles away, from their homes, at intervals dictated by financial and family circumstances—only to receive such brusque unwelcoming treatment from the professional staff that they gave up in despair.

Today we know that links with families cannot be thus dismissed. Very few children are today admitted as full-time patients in subnormality hospitals, and these numbers will grow progressively less.

But for those who are already adults in institutional care, every possible contact with the community must be maintained, family visits enjoyed on as informal basis as possible and the family welcomed as an integral part of the caring team.

WHERE ARE MENTALLY HANDICAPPED PEOPLE TODAY?

A very large group of mentally handicapped children and adults have always been cared for at home, and continue so to be cared for today.

If there is no additional physical handicap, parents may manage very well whilst the child is small, with support from health visitors, playgroups, nursery schools and special schools. The family with a handicapped member, though, always functions under a handicap—sleep is disturbed, visits outside the home are curtailed and family life is often severely affected. In some cases there is a breakdown of the marriage, and husband or wife—usually the wife—is left to carry on alone. If the breadwinner leaves, there is an additional economic burden, and without support the family will often decide that admission to an institution is the only solution.

A recent scheme has essayed to place children in foster homes, often with great success. The foster parents can be paid a salary to care for a handicapped child, a facility often denied to the natural parent.

Some imaginative schemes, often arranged by voluntary organisations, provide respite care—a break for the parents—by taking the child away for a short period. Some hospitals also provide short-term care for the child who is normally cared for at home.

There are privately run establishments, where the child has a home with other mentally handicapped children, and fees are paid by the parents, or in some cases by local authorities. These private homes vary greatly in size, staff and facilities, but since every child of school age must receive education, there is now more opportunity for those who provide residential care to make the establishment a home from which the child goes out for education. Some privately run homes have classes on their premises under the authority of the Local Education Committee.

Until a few years ago, many families with a mentally handicapped child did not have a holiday. Reluctant to expose the handicapped member to the curiosity or rejection of strangers, they remained shut away in their own home, seldom venturing out even for a day.

Fortunately, now, many hotels and boarding houses actively welcome families with handicapped members. Special holidays are available for mentally handicapped people of all ages, both from private homes and from hospitals and other residential establishments.

Group homes are being provided in many areas. In small groups —from four to five upwards—mentally handicapped people live together in ordinary houses, sometimes with a few special adaptations. They usually have some degree of supervision, even if it is only the interest of a neighbour. Such group homes are provided

B

by the Social Services departments of local authorities, and some hospitals provide a training facility, admininstered by the Health Authority, to prepare hospital residents for life in the community in a group home. At one time, the sexes were segregated as a matter of course, but increasingly, households are of mixed sexes, and the work of the house is shared suitably, as in an ordinary household.

Another form of residential provision is the hostel. Hostels vary greatly in size and staff. Some may be as small as a group home, with a staff supervisor, matron or warden in charge, and others may have as many as 40 residents, and a high proportion of staff to residents. Hostels are often provided for mentally handicapped people who are able to be employed—for example in sheltered workshops—or who can go out daily to a Training Centre.

Like the Group Home, the hostel is intended to provide a life-time home for the resident, so there will be clearly need to be an ever-increasing number of group homes and hostels to accommodate new residents from young people as they grow up.

Sheltered housing of various kinds is provided by authorities and by voluntary bodies. This type of amenity is sometimes intended for those who need more supervision than those who can live in group homes or hostels, and there are qualified resident staff who can give help at all times. In other cases married mentally handicapped people who want a degree of privacy are accommodated in specially built sheltered housing units.

Village communities have existed for a considerable time. These are self-supporting and provide for life-time care of mentally handicapped people. At present, most admit only those able to make some contribution, however small, to the life of the community. Crafts and rural skills are often the basis of the work of the community and products are sold to help the budget of the village. The staff are often well qualified professionals, teachers, instructors, nurses. Some have medical advisers and psychologists resident in the village. For some parents this type of provision fulfills all their requirements. Others cannot contemplate the separation involved, and prefer to keep their child at home as long as they themselves live. There are long waiting lists at most village communities, even for those considered suitable on the selection procedure.

Hospitals still provide residence for a very large group of mentally handicapped people today. In 1978 there were calculated to be approximately 50,000 adults and 4,000 children resident in hospitals. The concept of hospitals and their role is changing, but it is certain that a high proportion of those in hospital today will still be under hospital care, albeit care of a different type, and perhaps no longer called 'hospital' at all, ten years from today What we are concerned with is how best to use this period for the ultimate benefit of residents.

We have seen how the subnormality hospitals came to be built, and why they are so large. Both their location—remote from the community and often further isolated by high walls, gates, and extensive grounds—and their size have made the problems of introducing modern concepts of care most difficult. In the mid-1950s a number of Associations of Friends of Hospitals, parents and other well-wishers, began a movement to interest those outside the hospitals in the care and needs of both patients and staff. Hospital Friends Associations can do much more than simply raise funds for needed amenities, and today some are effective watch-dogs and pressure groups, helping to achieve recognition of good work, financial backing and changes in administration, as well as highlighting areas of concern.

ATTITUDES

Personal

We hear a great deal today about the need to change attitudes to mental handicap, particularly the attitudes of medical and nursing staffs. We hear very little analysis, however, of how our current systems of care *impose* negative attitudes upon people who may have begun their work among the mentally handicapped people with very positive ideas. For the very large majority of people entering a caring profession do so because they are already motivated by compassion and a desire to help those with whom they work. A few of course may be primarily concerned with career prospects, status, salaries, but these, in general, are preoccupations which arise later, and harden only as the emotional satisfaction of their work lessens.

Some of those staff members who have retreated into an apathetic acceptance of the status quo need, not so much an attitude *change* as a renewal of their original attitude and a chance to achieve some of their objectives of caring which will bring satisfaction. That is, they need a change in their working conditions.

New entrants into the field of care of the mentally handicapped look to those senior to them in experience for guidance and training. All too often they meet with neither. If this happens it is as well to remember that the responsibility for the daily opportunity to help those who need it is an individual responsibility not a collective one. There is always something you can do, and your duty is to inform yourself of all the tools available to you. Your own attitude is what eventually counts, both to you and to those you wish to help.

Public

Community attitudes have taken a long time to develop, and frequently take a long time to change.

Fear of those who are mentally handicapped is instinctive, and is reinforced when the mentally handicapped are kept shut away from others.

Largely due to the work of organisations such as parent-oriented bodies like the National Society for Mentally Handicapped Children, the whole question of mental handicap is now openly discussed. Public attitudes are still being formed, we are in a period of change. We are moving slowly into a greater public awareness of the size of the problem, of the particular difficulties of families and, most importantly, of the difference between mental illness, often curable, and mental handicap, a condition not amenable to medical cure, but capable of great improvement.

Children who are handicapped mentally and/or physically

are now taught, in some areas, in school with other ordinary children. The Act* which made this possible was passed in 1970—but not all Education Authorities have yet provided all the facilities envisaged by the Act, or extended all the facilities to mentally handicapped people which they already provide for others, such as full Further Education courses, though some Education Authorities have imaginative courses, both full and part-time. Attitudes to continued education for mentally handicapped people have yet to be generally set.

Parental

You will certainly quickly be told that some parents are 'over-protective' or that some caring staff have a similar attitude. It is important that one considers carefully the label 'over-protective', which in itself implies a judgement on the behaviour of someone else. Protective attitudes to those considered less able—very young children, old people, sick people, handicapped people—are very proper human responses.

The protective attitude of a parent indeed is instinctive—dictated by survival needs. Without such an attitude few infants, handicapped or not, would survive. If the period of helplessness, or relative inability for self-help, extends beyond infancy, it is natural that the protection by the parent will also be prolonged. The difficulty arises when, because of daily confrontation with a situation, the parent becomes unable objectively to evaluate the continuing need for protection.

The child grows, his experience of the world about him contributes to maturity, his experiments and their success or failure help him to learn. But if a mentally handicapped person, from any cause, well-intentioned or otherwise, is prevented from learning, from exposure to new experience, he will become further handicapped. So parents need to be helped to decide when to relax some of their care, how and when to introduce new learning, and this lesson has also to be learned by those who fill the role of parents by daily work with mentally handicapped people.

Such help will not make the work of parent or helper easier.

* Education (Handicapped Children) Act 1970.

On the contrary, it will often make it much harder, and it is often resisted for this reason.

To do something for a person is often much quicker, gives a better result, gives more satisfaction to the helper. To help a person to do something for himself transfers that sense of achievement from you, to him. Independence begins, and for some parents and helpers their own self-valuation as a needed and essential person begins to be eroded.

A compromise is essential. Parents and helpers need always to be *friends* of the mentally handicapped person—need to feel that they are wanted and appreciated; they will then have much more to offer than the simple authoritarian protective role.

Care staff should try to reinforce the concern and interest of parents, not deny it, and avoid value judgements of parental attitudes expressed by such statements as 'over-protective' or 'doesn't care'.

The best attitude is one which sees the situation as it affects the mentally handicapped person, and attempts to adjust the balance by providing for increased independence for those who need it, and increased care and love for those who do not receive it elsewhere.

Professional

There is another large area of concern in relation to attitudes, which may take much longer to change. Professional and craft bodies have grown up largely on an exclusive basis, believing that specialised skills, learned through many years of study or practical experience, should not be freely shared with others who have not served this long apprenticeship.

In early times, there were only two groups of people, clergy and laity, those who could read and write—the clerks—and those who could not. As learning was the prerogative of the clerks, they naturally became the most respected section of society and took over the most prestigious role—that of the priest. The priest-hood had, and has today, rites and mysteries jealously guarded. With the emergence of larger organised groups a second profession —the law—was organised, and as the arts of healing were handed down by the written word as well as by practical instruction, the profession of medicine began.

Gradually, many groups formed into united organisations, with a commonly accepted code of training and practice, with penalties for those members who did not provide services or goods at the agreed standard. From these guilds of craftsmen, modern trade unions and professional organisations developed.

They undoubtedly improved the training of their members and thus immeasurably improved the services and goods provided. But they all carried also the principle of exclusivity and this legacy is a two-edged weapon.

A team approach to the care of the mentally handicapped has been made more difficult because many of the professions involved know little of the training, expertise and skills of others, and may even feel threatened by them.

Teachers know little of the content of the three-year nurse training programme, for example, and nurses may know even less of the work of teachers. The same mutual ignorance applies to para-medical professions : occupational therapy, speech therapy, physiotherapy, remedial gymnastics, psychology, dietetics, pharmacology, among others, all play an important part in the whole care of mentally handicapped people, yet the expert in one field may know nothing of the skills of others.

So highly specialised is all this knowledge today that it would be impossible for each worker to absorb very much outside his own field. What is needed is a mutual respect for the knowledge and expertise of all those who form the care team, and, above all, *skill-sharing*—not *skill-hoarding.*

There are simple techniques, designed, planned, and programmed by specialists, which can be effectively carried out by non-specialists, without in any way eroding professional skills or reducing professional status.

The attitude here should be, if it will help, let's do it *together.*

CAUSATION

When a baby is born mentally handicapped, the first question the parents ask, aloud or to themselves, is 'Why?—how did this happen, why did it happen to me?'

Observers have noted that the reaction to the birth of a handicapped child to parents who had joyfully anticipated the birth of their baby is comparable to the grief of bereavement. This distress is often followed by a realisation that, unlike the finality of death, the pain and bitter disappointment will be a lifelong state. Parents react to this situation differently, but almost all ask 'Why?'

Sometimes the answer is known, and can be given to the parents at once, so can reassure them that future babies will probably not be affected. Sometimes the answer is less exact, and sometimes the only answer is 'we don't know'.

What is known, at present, is that there are probably some main groups of causes.

Genetic factors

These are inherited conditions, some of which may be present in healthy carriers—that is parents who do not themselves have the condition, but may pass it to a child.

The condition known as phenylketonuria is an example. Untreated babies develop severe mental handicap, and the cause has only recently been discovered. The condition is revealed by the presence in the urine or the blood of phenyl-pyruvic acid, discovered by a simple routine test.

Children who have a positive result to this test will be given a special diet throughout their childhood, and will then escape the effects, which are due to an inability to break down proteins.

There are genetic causes for other conditions, including some forms of cretinism and microcephaly, but these are rare conditions.

Chromosomal factors

The normal person has 46 chromosomes in 23 pairs in the nucleus of each body cell, of which half are inherited from each parent. These chromosomes carry the inherited characteristics.

If a baby is born with an extra chromosome he will be mentally handicapped. The most common form of chromosomal abnormality is mongolism, described by Dr. Down, and named after him, Down's Syndrome.

There are some other conditions caused by abnormalities of the chromosomes (Klinefelter Syndrome is a rare example), and as the science of cell genetics advances more will be known about their effects.

Infections

It has been known for some time that the unborn child may be affected by some illness of the mother, notably rubella (German measles), meningitis and tuberculosis.

The effect on the child is particularly disastrous at certain stages of development. Rubella in the mother in the first 12 weeks of pregnancy can cause deafness, blindness and mental handicap to the child.

Birth injuries

If the infant is deprived of oxygen at the time of birth, or receives an inadequate supply through delayed birth, forceps damage, or malposition, damage to the brain cells will result and may be so severe as to produce profound mental retardation.

Environmental factors

Increasingly we are discovering that substances which have become common in everyday life—lead in petrol, toxic wastes from manufacturing processes, food additives—are capable of producing effects upon unborn children as well as those exposed to such hazards in the community.

Prematurity

Very small babies are also at risk of mental handicap, especially if the prematurity is associated with a lack of ante-natal care or inadequate attention at birth. Very small premature babies are at risk of jaundice, which, if severe, can also result in brain damage.

RESEARCH

Modern technology, in particular the use of the electron microscope and new laboratory methods, has made it possible to study living cells, and to give answers to some questions of heredity, evolution and development.

The most profound contribution research has made in the field of mental handicap has been the identification of certain conditions whilst the baby is still at a very early stage of development in the womb. This is done by examining a sample of the fluid which surrounds the embryo foetus. The procedure is called amnio-centesis and can identify some conditions carried by the chromosomes, enabling the decision to be made whether the child shall be aborted, or carried to term.

Many considerations will influence such a decision, and the parents have an awesome burden if it is left to them to decide.

Investigation of all foetuses thus aborted continues to ensure that the findings of the laboratory are correct.

There are other methods of prediction of the chances of parents producing a mentally handicapped child, such as the newer science of dermatoglyphics, which can predict the possibility of the birth of a mongol baby by the study of the patterns of finger prints and foot prints of both parents. This work is still being expanded and already reveals other inherited tendencies.

SECTION THREE

The Mentally Handicapped Person

Developmental Diagnosis
  Key ages:
                 at birth
                 4 weeks
                 4–16 weeks
                 28 weeks
                 40 weeks
                 One year
                 1–5 years
Continued Development

Perceptual and Sensory Deficits
  Sight
  Hearing
  Confused reception
  Movement
  Touch
  Taste
The Team Approach

Definition of Needs
  Standard tests:
  Stanford Binet
  Wechsler
  Draw a man
  Illinois
  Vineland
  Gunzburg
Individual Programmes
  Example of Programme.
  Principles of Programmes

The Mentally Handicapped Person

We have spent some little time now talking about mental handicap in general terms : how handicap is defined, what may have caused it, how can it be prevented, but it is far more important for those who are to help the handicapped child or person to observe, to record and to understand each individual. Like the rest of the population, handicapped people will have some characteristics in common with each other, and we can look at these first.

All mentally handicapped people will be slower in understanding than the rest of us, and most will also be much slower in physical development. The result of this slowing, or retardation, will be that their achievements may not match their chronological age.

We shall discuss this also in more detail in the relevant chapters, but, for example, most babies can sit without support for a short while by the time they are six months old, most children are continent of urine by the age when they commence school at five years, most young adults can make social adaptations to different surroundings and can make decisions based on past experience. Mentally handicapped people are much slower in achieving normal milestones, and this slowness is related to the degree of their handicap.

To build bricks one upon the other requires co-ordination of the muscles of the eye and those of the fingers, hand and arm, all functions dictated by the brain. The usual age for this ability to begin is about 16 months, because by this age the baby's brain has developed sufficiently. But very profoundly retarded adults may not be able to perform even this simple action, and unless it is understood that they have not reached that stage of development, a full understanding of their need cannot be reached.

It is, however, wrong to base the treatment of a mentally handicapped adult, however severe his handicap, upon that appropriate for a baby. A man of thirty years with the mental age of a child of six, is nevertheless a man with thirty years of experience, however limited; and he will have hopes and fears, however ill-expressed, appropriate to those thirty years, and not to a six-year-old.

So the needs of each person need to be met. All mentally handicapped people, for instance, will need companionship; loneliness is not the prerogative of the intelligent. They need to be listened to, as they try to express their individual needs and thoughts. For those who are helping them, this means time and endless patience.

They need to have a sense of achievement, to be enabled to perform something for themselves by their own effort; and this, too, will require imagination and ingenuity from their helpers. It may take many weeks to show a mentally handicapped young girl how to arrange her own hair, if she is physically capable of doing so; but it will mean very much more if she achieves the result herself than if it is daily performed for her by others.

They need approval, just like everyone else. Praise for actions performed, and praise for the effort of trying; and the reward of approval can be shown as well by a smile, by the time given by those around them, as by more usual marks of approval such as sweets and treats, though these too have a place.

They need help to achieve social acceptance, by copying the social behaviour of others even if they do not understand it. They often behave instinctively (natural behaviour), embracing and kissing those they like, and reacting violently towards people and circumstances they do not like. We have to help them to suppress instinctive behaviour, so that they can mingle with others and not be rejected.

These are some of the mental and emotional needs of all mentally handicapped people, and in addition they will need help with physical functions.

Many of their movements are clumsy and awkward. They may have a shambling gait and poor posture, due to their poor muscle tone and poor co-ordination. If they are not stimulated by agreeable forms of movement, or by an interesting environment which encourages exploration, their physical condition will further deteriorate and may even result in total immobility. Whatever degree of movement is possible should be fostered and built upon by regular exercise.

Poor muscle control results in difficulties of speech and vision and affects eating and drinking. It may take great patience to teach a mentally handicapped child to feed himself, but if it is at all possible it must be done.

Poor muscle control may also result in delayed continence of bladder and bowel, and this may be further inhibited by the failure to understand the physical signals of a full bladder or bowel, or to understand the need to use the lavatory. Great patience, persistence and a calm approach to a standard routine may replace understanding by a trained response to the signals of the body.

So the picture of the mentally handicapped person emerging from our knowledge is one of an adult, with many childlike characteristics and some childlike behaviour, with immature responses to much of which goes on around him, with slower reactions and a slower rate of learning than normal and with certain additional needs specific to himself. The causes of his condition may be known or unknown, and the help he receives today may be greatly increased in future by new discoveries, for the frontiers of knowledge are expanding daily.

DEVELOPMENTAL DIAGNOSIS

We have so far discussed only the obvious signs of mental handicap and the treatment and help available in general terms.

As we now know that each mentally handicapped child or adult needs an individual programme designed to supply his specific needs, we have available a wide variety of tests which will identify these needs.

Assessment is essential for the proper analysis of individual needs, but it must always be remembered that this is the true purpose of such testing—assessment without the supplying of services designed to fulfil discovered needs is pointless.

It must also be remembered that in the cause of scientific accuracy, many tests must be carried out in controlled conditions, that is, under conditions as nearly the same for each person tested as possible. Under these circumstances the results can be compared with a known average, arrived at by the results of a very large number of similar tests. Thus we can know, for example, that in controlled test conditions the average time taken to carry out a task, or the standard achieved in carrying out a task, will be within certain limits the same for most people. Variations from the average will tend to show that the person tested is more able, or less able, in the particular activity being tested.

Individual performance of a test will also vary, due to many factors. The person may be 'off-colour', not absolutely fit at the time of the test, may arrive after an upsetting incident, may be alarmed by some factor new to his experience, by strange buildings, uniforms or a different staff member administering the test. In such cases those caring for a mentally handicapped person may hear that under test conditions, he has failed at some activity which they know can be performed perfectly well at home, or in the ward. Equally, sometimes, under test conditions, better performances is elicited, and an increased potential is discovered.

We will start by describing the earliest tests, which do not depened upon the co-operation of the person, and which are carried out very early in life to identify infants who may be mentally handicapped.

As in other tests, the baby is being tested against a normal average, against actions which most babies can perform at a given age.

If it is early discovered that the baby cannot perform some of the actions and behaviour at the important milestone or key ages, some immediate therapy can be given.

So what are the key ages?

At birth

The first one, of course, is the very moment of birth. As he leaves the womb the child must breathe for himself, his blood will no longer circulate through the placenta into his mother's blood stream, he must adjust to changes of temperature, perform his own excretory functions and obtain food by his own efforts as he sucks.

A tremendous adjustment—and one which, in sheer magnitude, will never again be matched in life.

Those around the baby at the moment of birth will be concerned with the most vital functions of independent life : can the baby breathe, move and cry ? Delay in any of these functions is critical, and if the delay is more than a few minutes, a record of the fact will appear on the medical note, and form the first indication of a deviation from the average.

The time taken to establish feeding is also critical. The baby is losing body fluid as he exhales air from his lungs, excretes from bowel and bladder, and perspires. He has only a limited store of body fluids and unless these are quickly replenished he will die. Healthy babies demand food by vigorous screaming and satisfy themselves by vigorous sucking. Delays in these activities are also noted.

Movements by the new baby follow a common pattern. They are unco-ordinated, the limbs flail about without purpose; he kicks, flexing and extending his legs and his small fists are tightly clenched; he will grasp a finger firmly if one is presented to him, an achievement which gives great delight to a new father, unaware of its instinctive origin.

He opens his eyes, and closes them quickly if light is too bright. Bright light will often provoke a sneeze. He jumps at sudden sounds and cries if the sound is particularly unexpected—but as everything is new, everything is unexpected.

Already an assessment of the baby is made, he can breathe, is active, responds to sound and light, feeds.

4 weeks

By four weeks of age other signs of development are present. He will now fix his gaze for a brief time on the face of his mother, or on a toy or other object if it is close to him. If he is placed in a sitting position and supported his head will fall forward. Placed on his face, lying down, he will turn his head to the side so that he can breathe freely. Feeding habits are established and he still demands feeds during the night as well as by day. He will quietly accept known sounds, such as the tinkle of a bell, recognise sounds associated with pleasure his mother's voice as feeding time—and still react by jumping or crying at loud or unusual sounds.

He will make small sounds, unassociated with crying, but these will not involve the lips and tongue as in babbling, which comes later.

His birth weight, which may have fallen in the period immediately after birth, will be regained and surpassed by several ounces.

4–16 weeks

In this period an awareness of the people and the world about him develops. He explores his clothing, blankets and cot with plucking movements, and examines his own fingers and toes, placing objects in his mouth for identification.

Placed face downwards he now lifts his head momentarily. He may fix objects with his regard more often, and for longer, and he will follow a moving object in his field of vision with his eyes.

He will show pleasure by a smile, and may begin to coo or babble, making sounds using his lips and tongue. He will enjoy water and kick and splash in the bath. Sudden noises will still elicit a scream, so will delayed meals and tastes he does not enjoy. He will show discomfort if he is not attended to when wet or soiled.

28 weeks

By this period the baby can sit briefly, and if supported, can hold his head steady. He will grasp toys and hold them for a short while. He will reach for objects and transfer them to his mouth or to the other hand. He turns quickly to the source of a sound and enjoys looking in a mirror. He knows strangers from family and friends and enjoys his meal times and the familiar routines of the household.

40 weeks

He can now sit alone and hold his head up strongly. He can build one brick upon another, feed himself with a spoon or rusk, make recognisable sounds such as 'mama', 'dada', pull himself to his feet by levering against a firm support, crawl and may clamber upstairs on his knees.

Not only is he aware of his surroundings, he shows that he is by waving goodbye, patting friends or animals, and always exploring by fingers and hands, everything about him.

One year
He can now stand and may begin to walk if one hand is held, and he is rapidly developing towards the goal of independent upright movement. He can grasp objects easily, but has still some difficulty in releasing them, so picks up and drops things many times, rehearsing this activity.

He will have two or three recognisable words, one may be a 'thankyou' sound for food or toys handed to him, one will certainly be 'no', and he will feed himself.

He will look at himself in a mirror and play with the reflection, he will look at pictures and show appreciation of them, he can pull objects and load a small cart of toys.

From 1 year to 5 years
Development continues and if there have been doubts about the child's performance at any of the key ages in his first year, much more intensive testing will now begin to discover if his backwardness is due to deafness, blindness, physical disability or mental disability.

CONTINUED DEVELOPMENT

We have spent some time describing the child in the first year of life because the brain develops at a faster rate at this age than ever again.

It is also important to realise that the body cannot carry out actions *in advance of the maturity of the brain*. If this is clearly understood much unhappiness will be avoided in the management of severely retarded children and adults. No-one expects a baby of four weeks to stand up and walk. Quite apart from the physical ability to do so; the brain centres concerned with complicated movement, with awareness of surroundings, and of self, are not developed. Similarly, many actions are beyond the ability of severely mentally handicapped children. But even if these children cannot initiate certain actions by themselves, they may be trained to perform them, using the experience of movement and of conditioned responses to replace normal responses. To explain this in more detail, normal infants and children are impelled by natural curiosity to explore the world about them and their own capabilities. They creep through gates, turn on taps, imitate the actions they have seen others perform, and indulge daily in activities which increase their knowledge and understanding of their surroundings. There are other actions which are imposed upon them, which the child himself would not instinctively wish to do, such as using the lavatory, washing his hands, dressing himself.

Some of these actions are repeated so often by the parents or family members that they become automatic, that is they are now 'conditioned responses'. The simplest example is answering a bell : a door-bell or a telephone. This conditioned response becomes so strong that few adults can listen to a telephone bell ringing without feeling impelled to answer it. But we were not born with an instinct to answer bells—this reaction is a learned one.

There are many such actions, achieved without special training by a normal child, which have to be taught to a mentally handicapped child, repeated and repeated until the action becomes automatic; and the same is true of mentally handicapped adults.

For instance, one thing that may need to be taught is a form of greeting. Normal adults will greet friends and strangers with some generally accepted social gesture : embracing, saying 'Hello', smiling, raising a hand. Small children often greet people by kissing or embracing, in imitation of adult behaviour towards them.

But some mentally handicapped adults remain unable to distinguish between forms of greeting which are appropriate, and those which are not : they may kiss and attempt to embrace strangers, and thereby cause embarrassment. They can, however, be trained patiently to greet others in a standard fashion : by offer-

ing a hand, saying 'Hello, how are you?' This will make it easier
for them to be socially accepted, because they are using a form of
behaviour expected of them.

Such behaviour, however, is not spontaneous and the mentally
handicapped person will still not be able to judge whether it is
suitable in a particular situation or not—like the small child
using a very adult expression in imitation of his parents, who risks
being laughed at or reprimanded according to the expression
used.

Developmental diagnosis, then, helps to establish in early childhood whether special needs exist for which individual help is
required.

PERCEPTUAL AND SENSORY DEFICITS

We have avoided the use of technical jargon as far as possible but
since some terms are in common use, we should know that the
adjective 'sensory' is used to describe those functions which depend
on the use of the senses; that the term 'sensory in-put' is used to
define the impression made upon us by objects and people about
us, and that the word 'stimulus' is used to mean anything which
produces a response.

We all acquire our knowledge of the world about us from the
evidence of our senses : sight, sound, touch, taste and smell. To
these physical senses we add an instinctive or intuitive 'sixth
sense', which we appear to inherit in varying degrees.

Mentally handicapped people may have reduced ability in
some of these areas, and there will be different levels in each of the
sensory areas, just as there are in individuals in the rest of the
population.

Some of us can clearly distinguish between colours, and would
never be confused between red and green. People who suffer from
colour blindness cannot make this distinction.

Partially sighted people may see colours as blurs of different
intensity; and we have only to look at paintings by some famous
artists to see how differently we all see the world about us.

It is fairly simple to understand that mentally handicapped

people can see, feel objects, listen and smell, because we can observe their reactions to stimulation of these senses. Many mentally handicapped people love musical sounds and show their pleasure when music is played, they often also love rhythm and will try to make corresponding movements. We are not so easily able to discover the *level* of perception, or their capacity to make sense of the information received via the senses.

It may help to remember the difference between sense and perception if we say 'I see you smile, and I perceive, therefore, that you are happy'.

Perception in this example involves a deduction on the basis of something seen.

You will need to understand that all mentally handicapped people have some defects of perception, and that these defects are always relative to their mental capacity. The task of those who are helping them is to analyse the defect and attempt to compensate for it by an individual programme of daily reinforcement, and where necessary, by technical aids.

Defective sight

A very high proportion of severely mentally handicapped people have impaired vision. Because the sense of sight is so important a stimulus to the brain, every opportunity to improve poor vision must be made.

Appropriate eye-testing by an ophthalmologist or optician may be difficult as very retarded people may not be able to understand and co-operate with the tests, but it is possible to make an estimate of their needs by observing how they look at objects. Do they need, for example, to bring things very close to their eye in order to focus? Can they recognise familiar people and objects at a distance? How minutely can they distinguish between one person and another, one object and another?

If there is any degree of sight impairment, all the ordinary commonsense aids should be employed; good lighting, clear bright colours on everyday objects, simple outline symbols for identification of essential equipment, as well as the provision of spectacles where appropriate.

Children with defects of gross motor movement who may be immobile for long periods of each day, need to be specially encouraged to use their eyes as a means of stimulation. Give them interesting moving objects to look at such as mobiles, and place them where they can see the movement of leaves in the wind or light reflected upon water.

Adults, too, who are less mobile need to be able to use their eyes, to be able to watch moving traffic, for example.

The television screen however must be used with caution. For reasonable periods the movement and colour will stimulate and interest the viewer, particularly if the activity is something which especially interests him—puppets and animals for younger children, horses, football or domestic activity, but the practice of seating mentally handicapped children or adults before a television screen as a means of filling the day is wholly bad. It can further damage sight where this is defective, and it results in apathetic boredom. Further, we have as yet little knowledge of, how much distress may be caused by the constant assault on the mind of those who cannot say 'switch it off'.

Every opportunity to see new things should be taken, and outings and holidays especially give the chance of new visual experience. Even those who are so severely handicapped that they are confined to bed need to be moved, so that they may see their surroundings from new angles and be aware of the changing seasons.

Defective hearing

Where sight is poor, hearing may become more acute to compensate. Some mentally handicapped people also have defects of hearing, and these are sometimes easier to discover than defects of sight. When sudden noises do not elicit any reaction, or a person does not respond to the sound of his name, of a bell ringing or the preparations for a meal, it is obvious to any observer that something is wrong.

Standard audiological tests are carried out by placing earphones over both ears, feeding in sounds at gradually increasing volume to each ear in turn and noting the level at which the sound is heard. But some degree of co-operation from the person being tested is needed, and the observations of those who are in daily contact with the handicapped person will be needed as well as the results of a test if the degree of mental handicap is severe.

If the person is capable of using a hearing aid, the problem can be overcome. Difficulty arises when there is so little mental capacity that hearing aids are thrown off and damaged.

Help can be given to a person with some hearing if those about him try always to gain the full attention of the handicapped person, always sitting directly in front of him and ensuring eye-contact before beginning to speak.

Deaf people have great difficulty in locating sounds, and this difficulty is present even when one ear has normal hearing.

Try to provide a quiet environment for learning for partially deaf people. In an attempt to stimulate the sense of hearing, for example, it is of little use to use teaching aids in a noisy room, as the background noise becomes an indistinguishable babel.

Confused reception

Stimulation is essential for the development of intelligence, and is supplied by his changing environment from the time a normal infant is born. In ordinary family life everything is new to the infant, he is continually stimulated by everything which is going on around him and his brain is accepting, sorting and making coherent conclusions every day. The experiences of his daily life are generally well ordered—water from a hot tap burns so it must be used with care, the sound of china and cutlery clinking means a meal, and so on.

A mentally handicapped child receives all the same information from his environment, *but* it does not make the same sense. It cannot be sorted and comprehended into cause and effect, and even less into the basis for future learning.

The nearest we can approach to an understanding of what it may feel like to be severely handicapped is to imagine that we are listening through ear-phones to four or more radio channels at once, unable to make sense of any of them; or that we are seeing the world from a merry-go-round turning at speed, and everything is turning so fast that familiar landmarks cannot be distinguished; or that we have arrived in a strange country where nothing relates to our previous experience and we can make order out of nothing that is going on around us. But we do not *know* how the limitation of intelligence affects mentally handicapped people, how they see our world or what their own inner life means to them.

We must give them every opportunity to make whatever degree of order and understanding of the world they can achieve, and we do this by discovering what they can perceive of their surroundings, and strengthening and reinforcing these perceptions so that they can be developed and improved.

Movement

After sight and sound, movement is essential for stimulation. However severe the physical handicap there will be some small degree of movement possible. Mastery of one movement, such as raising the head, leads on to other movements as the muscles strengthen. The stages of movement described for the infant and child in the first year of life are the basic movements, and should be worked upon first in the care of severely handicapped persons.

If standing and walking unaided are not possible, wheelchairs must provide mobility: they should not be used simply to transport people through the routine of the hospital day. Moving about the environment, the corridors, gardens and grounds gives opportunity to increase awareness of the everyday world, and stimulates further the senses of sight and sound.

Planned exercise can develop unused muscles, and physiotherapy and remedial gymnastics can help even the most handicapped. The presence of a trained physiotherapist is essential in the initial planning of the programme, but movement exercises can be carried out by all the helpers as part of the daily routine. Movement needs to be pleasurable. The more able people will enjoy games and sports. Water gives support to the body and many activities can be carried out in the swimming bath more easily than on dry land.

Handicapped people should be introduced to the swimming

bath with some care, so that they learn to trust themselves in water and not to fear it. Once confidence is established, water play and water exercise will be enjoyed.

In the past, the limitation of movement suffered by severely retarded children used to produce crippling contractions of the limbs, which added to the handicap and which, after several years, proved impossible to correct. An exercise regime is now regarded as essential even for the most immobile.

Touch

The impression received by touching and grasping objects are also important for stimulation, and can be provided for the most severely handicapped. Small objects of varying textures and shapes can be placed in the hand, the fingers can be guided over the hands and face of helpers and associated with the name of the person or object.

No matter how simple the activity, it can be a basis for learning, give pleasure and interest, and serve as a means of communication. Such activities may appear to the helper totally valueless, but they need to be persevered with regularly nevertheless, for repetition brings familiarity, and, eventually, a response.

Taste

The mouth is a very sensitive sensory organ and the young child tests every object by placing it in his mouth. As other senses develop, he learns to use other methods of discriminating between objects.

Mentally handicapped children may continue to use mouth identification of objects beyond the age of infancy, and this should not be discouraged. Caution is needed to make sure that the activity is supervised, and that the objects are harmless and clean. Sweet tastes are almost universally enjoyed, and communication can be established by the association of a pleasurable taste —a sweet, a taste of honey—with the voice and presence of a helper in even the most profoundly handicapped child. Only when some link of trust is establshed can any other therapy be commenced.

It is important, when caring for the very profoundly retarded who are capable of being fed by mouth, to do everything possible to ensure that this activity is enjoyed.

Texture of food, temperature of food and its taste are important. But so also is the social aspect. Close contact is needed when a person is being fed, and the activity can provide communication and pleasure. Feeding should not be regarded as just a means of supporting life, but as an opportunity of sharing experience.

Mentally handicapped people may have difficulty in chewing and swallowing—time is needed for their slower reactions and feeding must proceed at their pace, with hot food kept warm throughout.

Heat and cold are also experienced by the mouth. Find out whether a severely retarded person enjoys ice-cream, for example, or hot chocolate and ensure that there is variety in the foods he is offered.

To summarise, we need to utilise every available sensory function to stimulate the very profoundly retarded person. We need to continue the activities already possible with the less handicapped, and to extend them. We need to use the ordinary routines of everyday living imaginatively as opportunities for learning and pleasurable experience as well to implement specialist programmes.

THE TEAM APPROACH

Effective use of all techniques of stimulation requires a commonly agreed programme.

It is actually harmful to the handicapped person if those caring for him are not agreed upon uniform treatment.

If a child spends part of his time in a special school either daily or as a resident, it is most important that routines carried out in the education programme should be continued on the same lines when he returns to his home or ward.

Even as simple an action as washing hands in a hand basin has to be taught to a mentally handicapped child, and may also have to be taught to an adult who is being trained in life skills preparatory to discharge into community life.

It is obvious that unless all professionals involved are aware of the techniques employed by each other, and of the equipment used by each, a common approach cannot be devised.

If we examine the simple activity of washing hands, the student needs for instance to distinguish between the hot and cold tap in any basin, not only in the one he is being taught with—that the position of taps may vary, that sometimes the tap is marked, sometimes not. Even the order of filling the basin, finding soap and towel, and emptying the basin again, is a complex routine for a mentally handicapped person to grasp. It is certainly quicker and more efficient to do it for him!

The team must together decide which self-help skills are to be taught; how the activity will be broken down into simple stages; how the stages will be advanced; how the activity, once mastered, will be supervised, and so on. Recording is very important, so that all can see how well the programme is working and whether modifications are needed.

The objective is the maximum degree of independence, coupled with increased confidence and self satisfaction of the person to be helped.

The helpers will need much patience and a real understanding of the value of self-help programmes, as well as an appreciation of the need for co-operation by all concerned.

The team may consist of the physician—who will help identify the physical and mental level of achievement which can be expected of the person, and indicate any condition, such as epilepsy, which may introduce special factors in the programme; parents, nurses or care staff—that is, those who are in close contact with the person and are aware of his personal likes and dislikes, levels of concentration and fatigue and other individual characteristics; specialist therapists, where appropriate—speech therapist, physiotherapist; a psychologist; and a teacher will all be members of a therapeutic team.

The individual programme will include planned periods of specific activity, such as a session at school, another with a speech therapist, meal times; and other less structured periods of relaxation and leisure. New experiences should be introduced gradually.

The handling of a mentally handicapped person needs to be consistent at all times, and the system of reward or disapproval common to all, if confusion is to be avoided. So in a residential situation, such as a hospital, regular conferences between all staff contributing to care are essential for the proper conduct of learning and behaviour modification programmes.

DEFINITION OF NEEDS

In order to discover the areas of need of a particular person, many different tests are made, and the results of each assembled to form a profile.

The principles behind this profile are easy to grasp. If a person has defective sight and this is his only disability, he probably needs spectacles. If, in addition, he is deaf or physically handicapped, he may need both a hearing aid and a walking aid or even a wheelchair. Thus a profile for such a person would not only distinguish the need, but also the *degree* of need. Severe sight defects might require training at a school for the blind, severe physical disability might need a wheelchair, very severe physical disability, an electrically operated wheelchair. Assessment of physical handicap, and its degree, mild, moderate or severe, is well understood, and the need to check all physical systems to discover which can be utilised to help the defective ones is also generally accepted.

But in the case of mental handicap the assessment is less simple, as the mental processes involved are more complex, involving the measurement of intelligence, fine motor co-ordination, symbol recognition, language and communication, competence in the performance of everyday tasks, and stages of development.

Standard tests

The more usual tests are : —

Stanford Binet. The most used IQ test. Can be used on children of two years up to adult life.

Wechsler Test. Two versions, one for children and one for adults, aiming to estimate general knowledge and performance.

Draw-a-man Test. Mainly used for younger children. The amount of detail the child puts into his drawing—hair, eyes, ears, feet and fingers—is a measure of what he has learned from his environment. The drawings are often highly individual and a few examples will show how much they can vary, even when drawn at the same age.

Illinois Test. Particularly designed to test language development. Speech and communication depend on many factors : opportunity to hear speech and to imitate, understanding what is said and relating it to events, and the degree of ability to symbolise, that is to use words to represent objects, actions, feelings and so on.

Vineland Maturity Test Scale. This is designed to check competence in life skills such as dressing oneself, feeding oneself, use of the lavatory, travelling alone, money management and so on. It gives an estimate of intelligence for adults.

Gunzburg Charts. A method of continuously evaluating levels of achievement. The charts are visual records of areas of deficiency, and chart progress as it is made, for instance after use of a planned programme.

INDIVIDUAL PROGRAMMES

If, as the result of tests, it is found that the infant, child or adult has special needs, an individual learning programme will be devised for him.

The first requirement is an accurate record of the present stage reached, so that the success or failure of the programme may be judged by the results achieved.

Next the areas of need must be defined and priorities decided upon. No one, handicapped or not, can learn everything at once, and everyone has a need for relaxation and leisure.

The programme must be strictly structured so that *everyone* in contact with the person understands it and carries it out in a similar fashion. Mentally handicapped people even more than others require continuity and uniformity in their learning programmes. They can become confused and bewildered by conflicting practices.

Professional knowledge is essential to the drawing-up of a programme. *BUT* not every activity on the programme needs to be performed by an expert. If a person has a speech defect, a speech therapist will initiate sessions and commence a programme to help; but everyone in contact with him can put into practice at every opportunity the principles suggested by the therapist. So everyone involved will need to understand the methods used.

Opportunities for speech improvement cannot be limited to one session a week in a clinic. All human contact offers opportunities for communication, and as long as we patiently repeat phrases and speak *to* not *at* mentally handicapped people, we can hope that some at least of what we say is being retained and slowly and painfully absorbed. We can never know how much. But we have evidence in *A Long Way to Manhood*, the story of her mentally handicapped son, written by Alice Candy, that even after years speech may be achieved. Mrs. Candy's son repeated phrases spoken to him by his grandmother many years before. This one small example illustrates that programmes which are apparently fruitless can still produce results if they are persevered with.

Similarly, an understanding of social attitudes, or the use of the lavatory, may take some individuals many months to achieve, particularly if they are adults who have not previously had the opportunity of education and learning programmes.

We have to make allowances for the slower rate of learning, the need for patient repetition to imprint the desired action on the mind of the mentally handicapped person, for his distractibility and the enormous effort he must make to fix his attention for any length of time on purposeful activity.

The individual programme, then, should be planned by experts, in conjunction with those in daily contact with the handicapped person, and, where it is possible with those of sufficient intelligence, with the handicapped person himself. This involvement of the handicapped person should be made whenever it is possible. Young adults in the moderately severely handicapped category will leave special schools with some skills already learned. They may be able to read at a simple level, to keep themselves clean and tidy, and to sew or garden. A continued learning programme for them is vital if they are not to regress to a lower level of ability, and this will have greatest hope of success if it takes into account the particular interests of the person for whom it is designed.

Structuring the programme simply means making very definite objectives, designing teaching practices and giving very exact instructions on how the practices should be carried out, when they should be done, how long each activity should last, how often repeated and how recorded. A record of the learning session and the result is essential.

As an example, let us suppose we wish to teach a child how to use a spoon, or drink from a cup, when he has never previously done so. First, we must not assume any knowledge. You have yourself used a spoon for so many years that you now pick it up, fill it with food, carry it to your mouth and eat from it and return it to your plate without thought.

Example of learning programme

To structure this activity we should plan a programme which commences with a linking of the activity to its purpose, thus :—

Sit down at the table with a dish of suitable food in front of the person under instruction. Sit in front of him, or beside him in such a way that you can see his face, and he yours. Place a spoon at the right hand (left if the person is known to be left handed). Say 'You are going to eat your pudding with a spoon today'.

Pick up the spoon yourself, notice the muscle movements involved both in picking up the spoon, grasping it and lowering and raising it.

Put the spoon into the hand of the child, reproducing the movements you know are involved. Keep your own hand over his to reinforce the movement.

Lower the spoon to the dish and show by the movements of

your own hand how food is loaded into the spoon, maintain the support of your hand. Describe in simple words what is happening —'We push the spoon into the pudding against the plate, then lift it up to our mouth, open the mouth, put the spoon in, lick the pudding off, take it out, put it down again for another spoonful', and so on.

You will already see how complex an activity an everyday action such as this can be to a very handicapped child, and how many patient efforts will be needed to master it.

The conditions for learning must also be carefully considered. It is suggested that to learn to use a spoon the activity of eating a sweet pudding is likely to produce best results. The child has already had some food, so he is not hungry—he wants to eat the pudding and is more likely to co-operate with an activity which has a desired result.

It cannot be continued to the point of boredom, because the pudding will be eaten, either with help at every stage or a gradually decreasing amount of help from the helper.

Principles of programme planning

This element of boredom or exhaustion with an activity must be taken into account in programme planning. If it is not, the learning will be rejected and future programmes jeopardised. Where repetition is needed, the planner of the programme should be able to estimate how often an activity can be safely repeated before boredom sets in, and those who work on the programme need to inform the planner if the student does become bored.

This may indicate readiness to move on to a further stage, or inability to master the activity in its present form. Either way, continued use of the activity is fruitless.

If we continue to look at the example above—teaching the use of a spoon—we can see that there are many other learning possibilities in the activity. It involves speech patterning—as one talks to the child repeating the same words clearly : spoon, pudding, hand, hold this, lift this, up, down. It also involves grasping skills, especially that of the index finger, used to identify the spoon and lift it, which skill can be reinforced by giving the child other

c

objects to hold and grasp, different objects with a variety of shapes, sizes and textures to develop the muscular co-ordination needed to use tools.

Breaking down a more complex activity, such as the use of the lavatory, will require much more structuring, and much more patience. There are published accounts of methods used in some institutions with good results (*Take Six Children*), but as all situations are different, an individual programme must be individually planned by those who will be in daily contact with the mentally handicapped person, who are familiar with the routine of his day and the amenities available and who have a realistic attitude to what is hoped for and what may be achieved.

Nothing at all will be achieved unless *all* those concerned are in favour of the activity and willing to carry it out systematically.

The rewards in terms of improved daily life for mentally handicapped people from such learning programmes are so great, and the relief to those who care for them in terms of unrewarding chores so valuable in time and energy, that it is an area to which all care staff, at every level, should give prior consideration.

If a mentally handicapped person can do something for himself, however small, or however seemingly difficult, be it combing his own hair, or cooking his own lunch, means must be found to enable him to do it.

SECTION FOUR

Basic Health Care
  Diet
    Overweight Diets
  Excretion
  Sleep
  Hygiene
    Skin
    Hair
    Feet
    Menstruation
    Masturbation
    Nasal Discharge
    Handwashing

Basic Health Care

Mentally handicapped people have the same needs as others, but in some areas they have special needs.

The slower metabolic rate which occurs in many conditions results in poor circulation, slower adjustment to temperature changes, also slower absorption of food.

Difficulties of muscle co-ordination make some movements clumsy, and as a result, fear of falling may render a handicapped person less willing to move freely.

Diet needs careful attention, and if there has been neglect in early life there may be damage to teeth which renders chewing difficult. Chewing food is important to the correct development of the jaw and alignment of the teeth, and to continue with a soft, bland diet too long will aggravate the difficulties.

Mentally handicapped people will need a temperature-controlled environment, adjusted for day and night; opportunities for exercise and movement; correct diet; cleanliness to give comfort to the body and reduce the risk of skin infections; and correct clothing and footwear.

DIET

A balanced diet contains the proteins needed to build body cells, fats which provide some of the heat-giving requirements, carbohydrates for energy and vitamins to complete the diet. Fluid is needed to transport all the nutriments around the body and to assist in excretion.

Mentally handicapped people often have a liking for very sweet foods and sweetened drinks, so they become overweight easily.

Tooth decay is more rapid when sweet items are eaten throughout the day, so that the sugar level in the mouth remains high.

Eating snacks between meals is a bad practice for anyone, and the regime for mentally handicapped people can be overloaded with biscuits, crisps and aerated drinks.

Breakfast is an important meal and should contain some whole fibre food (such as cereal, brown bread or bran), as well as protein (eggs, bacon, fish), and fluid (fruit or fruit juice, coffee, tea, milk or water).

Milk and dairy products are important for the health of teeth and bones, and one pint of milk daily should be given either as a drink or in other foods such as custards or soups.

If lunch is served around noon, there should be no need for mid-morning snacks, though fruit might be enjoyed then. Every attempt must be made to develop a taste for chewing such foods as apples, raw carrot and other shredded vegetables. Lunch meals should contain protein (meat or fish), vegetables and a pudding.

The last meal of the day should not be too early, so that the night is disturbed by hunger, nor so late that digestion is not complete before sleep. It should make up for any deficiences in the day's menu—for example, if insufficient protein is taken at lunch, the evening meal can contain meat, fish or eggs, or a vegetable protein such as beans.

The best diet is a varied one, so that all available foodstuffs are utilised and prejudices against certain foods cancelled out by others.

Overweight diets

It is very important to keep the weight of handicapped people, particularly the severely handicapped, within manageable limits. Too much fat will further decrease mobility, place extra strain upon the heart and make their daily care much more difficult.

If obesity is a problem, a strict diet watch must be kept, as part of a weight reduction programme. Very fat people often 'eat nothing' and only an accurate record of what is actually consumed in a day will reveal the exact intake.

In advising parents or others in the community on weight problems it is often useful to involve a group such as Weight-watchers, so that overweight people can receive the support of others as they deal with the problem. If no group is available, it is a good idea first to make an accurate estimate of food intake over a period of one week, and then suggest that the quantities of sugar, sweet drinks, biscuits and cakes be cut by half.

More success is obtained by reducing the amount in the first place than by attempting to cut it out completely. Mentally handicapped people may derive great pleasure from their sweet foods, 'pop' and ice cream. So if it is discovered in the preliminary check, for example, that they are having four glasses of 'pop' and eight biscuits during the day, a reduction to two glasses and four biscuits makes a good start.

In an institution, the daily diet will be planned to include all the elements of a balanced diet. It is the task of the helpers to see that those in their care accept the food offered, while on the other hand keeping a watchful eye on the extra foods taken as treats.

Parents often give extra food to a mentally handicapped member on his return from school or training centre, as a compensation for not providing food all day, and as a pleasure to be enjoyed together. If possible, try to advise parents that another pleasurable activity be substituted; or that non-fattening foods be substituted for sweet ones. There are many excellent books of such recipes suitable for all ages and stages, which also provide information on the healthy weight for people of different height and physique.

Children grow rapidly until puberty, usually between 12 years and 14 years, and in adolescence there is a second spurt of growth to maturity. In this period there is a primary need for adequate protein. In adult life the amount of food needed is relative to the energy output of the body : too little, and the person loses weight, becomes listless and unhealthy; too much and the person becomes fat.

EXCRETION

The end product of all foodstuffs, once the essential elements have been absorbed, is excreta.

The lungs filter the air and remove from the body the carbon dioxide produced by the metabolising of foods.

The bowel absorbs fluid from the residue of all foods and excretes the waste. The longer the food residue remains in the bowel, the more fluid is absorbed and constipation may result.

The kidneys filter all fluid and excrete unwanted substances in the urine, including the residue of any drugs taken.

The excretory functions are important to health and it is usually accepted that a daily evacuation of the bowel is normal. It is easy to become over-concerned with the function of the bowel and to give laxatives when attention to diet would correct the condition, but neglect to achieving a reasonable pattern can give discomfort to mentally handicapped people. Those responsible for their care should notice and record any difficulty and take such action as is needed.

More exercise, fruit, extra roughage and extra fluids will help constipation. Simple laxatives such as prunes, rhubarb and senna should be tried before the more potent drugs.

The use of the lavatory and toilet routines has also to be taught to mentally handicapped people, and if this training is commenced early and patiently repeated they will not have to suffer the added discomfort of incontinence.

SLEEP

Adequate rest is just as important for mentally handicapped people as others, and those who have experienced a sudden change in their lives—for example, leaving home, or being transferred to hostel or group home from hospital—may have their sleep pattern disturbed. Without the help of mild sedatives, lack of adequate sleep may cause confused behaviour and emotional upset.

Reports of failure to adjust to a new environment should always indicate an investigation into sleeping habits, and medical advice should be sought if sedation is needed.

Sleep requirements and sleep patterns differ among individuals and change with age. Nurses and helpers should be alert during the day for signs of undue fatigue or irritability which may indicate disturbed sleep.

HYGIENE

Skin

The skin is the largest excretory organ of the body and needs to be clean to function properly.

The sweat glands excrete fluid and also hormonal products. If the body areas are kept washed and dry, odours are minimised, but if perspiration is left on the skin, subsequent sweating will act upon the old excretion and produce an unpleasant smell. The acidity created by this process also allows bacteria to develop, which in turn produce infections such as spots and pimples which can become further infected and lead to boils.

The skin produces a natural oil which keeps the body surface supple. Harsh detergents remove this protection, allowing cracking and dryness to develop.

The object of skin care is to remove dirt without damage to the skin, and after washing, careful drying of the skin is needed. Bcause mentally handicapped people have a tendency to dry skin, or overactive sebaceous (oil-producing) glands, extra care is needed in washing and drying, and nurses and helpers should ensure that this need is understood by those capable of attending to their own personal hygiene.

Hair

Hair needs regular washing. The simplest types of shampoo available are probably mild soap, and the shampoos prepared for babies which do not irritate the eyes. It is important to make personal hygiene as pleasant as possible if it is to be performed regularly, and a stinging, smarting shampoo will certainly not encourage good routines.

Hairdressers can often suggest styles of cutting which are easy to manage and attractive. Both men and women need to be encouraged to be interested in their appearance.

Care of the feet is often difficult for retarded people, and if corns and ingrowing toe-nails develop mobility will be further impaired. Chiropodists may be able to advise on equipment to enable a handicapped person to clip his or her own nails, if scissors are a problem.

Menstruation

Menstruation is often difficult for girls to handle, so the use of sanitary towels and method of disposal must be carefully explained and demonstrated until it is understood. The importance of bathing or use of the bidet at such times must also be taught.

Masturbation

Adolescent males experiencing nocturnal emissions also need careful explanation of why this happens, and to be shown how to wash and change nightwear if necessary. Masturbating males may also need guidance on hygiene needs. If the helpers are not alert to these developments, severely retarded young adults may be exposed to unnecessary anxiety and discomfort.

Those who care for mentally handicapped people should be careful to display no attitude of censure or disapproval in their response to any natural biological function; only a desire to impart sufficient knowledge of generally acceptable behaviour to enable mentally handicapped people to function as well as possible in a social situation.

Nasal discharge

Some mucus production is essential to keep the nasal passages moist and able to filter the air on its way to the lungs. If the secretion is excessive, due to infection with the virus of colds or 'flu, or to mechanical damage—pushing beads or other small objects into the nose—discomfort results.

Infection of the nasal passages may result in a greenish-yellow purulent discharge, which spreads the infection into the surrounding skin, and sometimes up into the sinuses.

Running noses are a common sight in institutionalised children, and in some adults, and may be caused by too-vigorous wiping and blowing, which increases damage to the tissues.

The tissues of the nose are delicate and easily damaged. Running noses should be gently wiped, and under no circumstances should the nose be tightly held in a handkerchief when blowing. This forces infected mucus into the sinuses and aggravates the condition.

A little vaseline put gently into the nose at bed time will often relieve soreness during sleep. This can be done when the child is sleeping, if it is resisted. Vaseline will also protect the surrounding skin.

Medical advice should be sought for a persistently running nose. A purulent discharge must always be reported, as it may indicate more serious and communicable infection. But it is worth noting that it is quite often the most unloved child in a group who has the running nose. His running nose makes him still less lovable, and it is difficult to identify where the cycle begins. Comforting and gentle attention to the running nose may produce improvement.

Hand washing

The importance of handwashing after the use of the lavatory cannot be over-emphasised. Bacteria exist in the bowels of everyone. Each individual eventually adapts to his own bacterial invasion and they cause him no harm, but transmitted to others they may cause acute illness.

The group of diseases called 'enteric' can only be transferred by ingestion, that is by eating or drinking the toxic products of bacteria or viruses, excreted in faeces.

The most common method of transmission is by contaminated hands taking the infection to the mouth. Do not forget the hazard of the toilet flush levers, door handles and seats, which need regular disinfection.

Mentally handicapped people need a great deal of help to understand the need for thorough hand washing after use of the lavatory; so strict attention to cleanliness in toilets is needed by staff, who must also ensure that hands are washed again before meals, and that similar precautions are taken by themselves.

In any institution some common infections become a regular feature. They can only be contained by constant vigilance, and it is the duty of staff to ensure that they themselves do not pass on infections to themselves or others by lack of knowledge or attention to good practices.

Maintenance of body temperature

The normal temperature of the body is maintained by a delicate balance between heat production and cooling, provided by the circulation. Changes in the environmental temperature, extreme heat or cold, produce discomfort and if prolonged, exhaustion and physical breakdown (heat-stroke, frost-bite).

Even moderate changes may produce ill effects in immobile people who are unable to make personal efforts to help themselves.

Staff and helpers need to be alert to daily temperatures, provide heat or shade, protect residents from excessive sun exposure, cold winds and wet, and to ensure that clothing provided is appropriate. Natural fabrics, cotton and wool, are usually less irritant to sensitive skins than synthetics, allow better circulation of air to the body and have better absorptive and insulating properties. Chilling pre-disposes to infection and over-heating causes loss of body fluid, especially dangerous to young infants.

Room temperatures should not be below 70° F.

SECTION FIVE

Specialised Hospital Care

Physical Care

Food Hygiene

Bathroom Hygiene

Ward Hygiene

Sleep Management

Moving Immobile People

Severely Deviant Behaviour

Profoundly Handicapped People

Multiple Disability

Epilepsy

Autism

Liasion with Family and Community

Specialised Hospital Care

There has been a considerable reduction in the number of people admitted to subnormality hospitals in recent years. Many long-stay patients have been discharged, after some rehabilitative training, to live in hostels in the community, with or without supervision.

Children, in particular, are no longer admitted to hospital care as a life-time solution, just because they are mentally handicapped.

But there are still over 50,000 people of all ages in subnormality hospitals, and some of them will never be able to be discharged for a variety of reasons.

Some of these are people who are now aged or ageing and who are so severely handicapped, both mentally and physically, that they cannot adapt to life in the community. Others are multiply afflicted, perhaps by poor mobility, made worse by lack of suitable treatment when they were first admitted, by poor sight or hearing and by intractable incontinence. Yet others are of such low ability levels that they will always require more supervision than can be provided outside an institution.

For those who must continue to be cared for in hospitals, there have been very considerable changes already, and there will be many more in the next decade. The greatest change has been the acceptance of the need to see the environment of the mentally handicapped resident as his home, first, and only secondly as a hospital. This means that no more large units will be built, and in existing establishments, the accommodation is being divided into much smaller units by all means available.

The smaller unit requires much more staff to provide adequate supervision and support, so there will have to be a considerable recruitment to supply even the basic staffing needs dictated by the new concept of care.

In some hospitals, small groups of elderly women and men are accommodated in specially built homes and wards, equipped with comfortable living conditions much closer to the conditions provided by old people's homes in the community.

Some hospital accommodation is provided for those who go to sheltered workshop or training centres daily—their accommodation is like hostels for working people outside. Other hospitals have provided accommodation for married people and continue to give total support within a hospital setting.

Hospital schools, specially built and equipped and staffed by teachers from the Education Authority, may also be provided within the hospital grounds.

Some hospitals have built small hostel units where residents live for a while to be trained and prepared for life in the community by acquiring self-help skills of shopping and cooking, laundry and self care.

Innovation and experiment is bound to continue and no universal pattern of care will be found for hospital residents for some years.

Mentally handicapped people are usually admitted to subnormality hospital today for reasons which are mainly medical. Though there are still admissions for social reasons, and emergency admissions when family conditions change, the current philosophy is not to admit to hospital unless suitable care cannot be given outside a hospital.

There are some cases, where the effect of disability is so great that expert medical and nursing care is needed, in addition to all the other therapeutic care already described. These conditions are those where a profoundly disabling physical condition which requires life-supporting professional skills is superimposed on severe mental retardation.

There are for instance skeletal abnormalities associated with some forms of mental handicap : hydrocephalus (water distention of the skull), megalocephalus (greatly enlarged brain), microcephalus (very small brain). There are other conditions, such as gargoylism, where the deformity affects the bones of the face. Epilepsy in its most severe form—grand mal—will require hospital care as the fits threaten life through asphyxia, and careful medication is constantly required to reduce the number of fits.

Some severely retarded people with additional physical handicaps such as blindness, deafness, immobility, may need hospital care; and so may those with cerebral palsy, if they are also totally bedridden.

Behaviour problems of the more severe type, too, may necessitate hospital admission, and a programme involving both psychiatric (medical) care and psychological and social training may be needed for some time.

Intractable incontinence may make life outside a hospital so difficult as to be impossible.

About half the people at present in subnormality hospitals are able to perform some self-help skills for themselves. The duty of the nurse or helper is to identify those who have some ability, to decide which skills will give the greatest satisfaction to the resident, and to request expert help in designing a programme to acquire them.

The second responsibility is to provide opportunity to exercise the skill learned regularly, so that performance improves, and to be alert to the moment when a new skill can be achieved for further progress.

The nurse in a curative medical or surgical ward derives satisfaction from observing how medical skills enable a sick or diseased body to heal. In the field of mental handicap the nurse transfers this satisfaction to achieving a gradual and continuing improvement in the awakening and responding functions of a handicapped mind.

PHYSICAL HOSPITAL CARE

If we make a very rough estimate that half of the residents in a subnormality hospital will be able to achieve some degree of independence in living, we are still left with the half who for different reasons will not. These are the group who cannot sustain life without skilled nursing care, or whose quality of life will totally depend upon those who care for them.

It is possible to keep incontinent people reasonably clean and free from sores without any personal, caring involvement with them at all. After all, mothers of normal babies who have made a total emotional rejection of the child often nevertheless provide impeccable physical care. But we know now that without the loving and warm relationship usual between mother and child, no matter how well the child is fed, clothed and housed, that child will be a damaged person. So the first thing to remember is that cleanliness is not the most important requirement of all. But in a hospital it can be critical, because of the ever-present danger of spreading infection.

Nursing skills can do much to alleviate the problem. The time when micturation (passing urine) or evacuation of faeces (bowel movement) is most likely can be determined by careful observation, so that clothing and linen need not be soiled. There is for instance a reflex action of the colon after taking food or drink, or urine may be passed if taps are turned on. Each person will have an individual pattern.

Prompt attention to changing and cleaning will avoid soreness and smells, and nurses now have a wide variety of incontinence pads and appliances, skin oils and lotions, to make the task of cleaning residents more efficient.

The danger of cross-infection from excreta can be minimised by intelligent practices. Soiled linen and clothing should never be thrown on to the floor, or sorted in corridors. A closed container should remove contaminated items to the sluice rooms where they should be dealt with promptly. Staff should wear protective clothing whilst dealing with contaminated items, and wash thoroughly before undertaking any other duties.

Enteric diseases such as sonné dysentery, salmonella infections, are readily passed in institutions, and can become an intractable problem. So every attempt must be made to initiate a good programme of ward hygiene, and this should extend to day rooms and classrooms if incontinent adults and children use them. The sand pit and water play equipment are especially vulnerable to infections of this type. Efficient protective clothing for users who are liable to incontinence must be provided.

Some residents may have warning aids prescribed—electric devices to ring a bell or give other signals when urine is passed. Helpers and nurses need to attend to such signals promptly if they are to be useful.

Whenever possible try to ensure that severely retarded incontinent people cannot smear their excreta with fingers or hands, and thus transfer possible infection. Suitable clothing or nightwear may help.

Soap and water, sunshine and freely circulating air are powerful disinfectants and should be freely used, as well as specific chemical disinfectants, in the control of enteric diseases.

FOOD HYGIENE

Feeding and serving meals is another potential disease-transmitting hazard. In the hospital kitchen all precautions should be taken to ensure that the food reaches the residents in best condition.

Usual sources of contamination are the hands of catering staff, dirty utensils, improper storage of food at too high temperatures, contamination by insects or animals, re-heating of foods and, more rarely, food which is unfit for consumption.

Nurses should not only notice the quality of the food supplied, but should check on the serving equipment to ensure that it is clean and in good order.

Damaged and cracked crockery, serving containers which are not clean and sound are all potential dangers to the patient, who cannot protect himself. Food-borne infections can kill, and always result in pain and considerable distress.

Everything used to feed a helpless person must be spotlessly clean, and those residents able to feed themselves need to be helped to achieve a standard which will reduce spills and accidents.

Meals must be promptly cleared and trays and dining tables and equipment washed and cleaned as soon as practicable. Stale food items attract flies and other disease-carrying vermin. Handwashing before food cannot be too often stressed.

BATHROOM HYGIENE

In lavatories and washrooms there is a greater risk of transmitted disease than anywhere else.

Individual toilet items at least serve the function of limiting the spread of any infection from one person to another. So each resident should have his own toothbrush and mug or glass, face and body cloth and towel, stored with sufficient space between each owner's equipment to avoid touching. Toilet items need to be easily recognised by those able to help themselves, in different colours or with different symbols.

Lavatories need to be checked for cleanliness by nurses, who should also supervise personally the routine disinfection of flush levers, door handles and toilet seats. However efficient domestic helpers may be, they do not always have the training needed to identify potential hazards.

Cleaning equipment should not be carried from one area to another: mops and cloths and brushes used in lavatories and bathrooms should be used only there. It is not even advisable to use the same items for several units in an institutional setting.

If it seems that there is over-emphasis on the role of the nurse in this area, no apology is made. To be clean and comfortable and protected from preventable infection is the right of those who are not able to provide these conditions for themselves. They depend upon the knowledge and conscientious practice of the nursing staff to achieve these basic needs.

WARD HYGIENE

It is usual to provide a rather higher room temperature for mentally handicapped people than for others, because they very easily feel cold and uncomfortable in low temperatures.

This raised temperature, 75°–80°F, makes it all the more essential to provide a full circulation of air. Where air-conditioning is provided, the filters removing dust and droplets from the air need regularly changing. Where no system is installed, windows must provide adequate ventilation. This can be achieved by a programme of opening windows when most of the ward occupants are elsewhere, and ensuring that those confined to beds are warmly wrapped whilst the air of the room is changed, before closing the windows again. Some windows are designed to open to admit sufficient air without draughts.

Technicians are responsible for maintaining temperature control and air conditioning systems, and for ensuring that windows can be opened as needed. Nurses and care staff need to be sure that these functions are carried out efficiently for the benefit of the residents, and should regularly note ward temperatures and ventilation.

SLEEP MANAGEMENT

People who are in bed all day will need to have sufficient activity provided to avoid as far as possible sleeping during the day.

People on sedatives to control fits or involuntary movement will be sleepy at times, but for these, periods of day-time sleep should be kept as short as possible, to ensure a more acceptable night sleep pattern.

The preparations for the night need to be phased gently so that the activities of the ward are conducive to a restful period before the lights are turned low. It will soon be found which residents prefer darkness and which like a low light through the night, and it may be possible to adjust the beds' places to achieve the greatest comfort.

Very severely handicapped people may not be able to indicate when they are too hot, or too cold, or too uncomfortable to sleep. If they did not have the supper meal or drink for some reason, their sleep may be disturbed by hunger. All simple methods of achieving natural sleep should be tried before having recourse to drugs.

MOVING IMMOBILE PEOPLE

However physically handicapped, both children and adults need frequent position changes to avoid sores and contractions. Some spastic people experience pain in certain positions which is relieved when they are moved.

Very heavy people will need two or three people to change their position, but this must be done regularly, perhaps at the same time as a wash or a massage. Meal times too provide an opportunity for regular changes of position, both when preparing for the meal and when clearing away utensils and trays.

Apart from changes of position, immobile patients will need to be moved from one place to another. Every opportunity to move profoundly handicapped people should be used—to communicate with them, to refresh them, to give them a different view of their environment.

Changing the level of the bed or chair will enable them to see from a different window or through a different door, even in bad weather. In good weather every effort must be made to ensure that from a balcony or other sheltered place they can observe the trees and plants, traffic passing, and other people at work or play.

To condemn a profoundly handicapped person to the further sentence of imprisonment in one corner of a ward or room, day in, day out, is totally unacceptable. However small the change, it will improve his daily life.

SEVERELY DEVIANT BEHAVIOUR

It would be foolish to suggest that no mentally handicapped person exhibits deviant behaviour, but as this extreme condition requires psychiatric and psychological treatment it will always be dealt with by properly qualified staff in hospitals competent to manage such problems.

Indications for urgent intervention do not usually arise suddenly, and nursing and care staff will observe changes and deterioration in those they see daily before the consultants, who may be less familiar with the individual, do so. Attention should always be paid to reports by parents or residential care staff of behaviour changes which indicate a worsening state, so that problems can be dealt with before an acutely violent episode provokes disaster.

PROFOUNDLY HANDICAPPED AND MULTIPLY HANDICAPPED PEOPLE

There is often confusion in the minds of those unfamiliar with mental handicap about what is meant by the term 'severely', or 'profoundly' handicapped. This confusion is all the greater because it is possible for a person to be profoundly mentally handicapped whilst appearing, superficially at least, to be physically normal. Thus parents with children with very severe mental handicap who nevertheless look perfectly normal, are the ones who receive least sympathy and help from onlookers when the child behaves in a bizarre manner.

It is in a hospital that most people with very profound degrees of handicap, or with mental handicap associated with physical disability and deformity, are to be found. Nursing skills may well be pre-eminent in such cases, and may indeed be essential to preserve life. But it must also never be forgotten that for these people any hope of joy or pleasure in their life, however brief, is totally at the mercy of those who give daily care.

Fully professional service at the highest level of skill may be needed, for instance, to feed people totally unable to receive nourishment except by medical and nursing techniques. Movement and sensory stimulation may also be dependent upon professional helpers; and if further afflictions—blindness or deafness—are involved, it will require all the dedication and invention of staff to bring some quality of human enjoyment to the lives of this, admittedly small, group of mentally handicapped people. Yet it is working with this group which gives the helper, usually the nurse, with a strong sense of dedication the greatest satisfactions.

This type of care is immensely demanding and staff in these units will require more than average opportunities for change and refreshment of spirit. On the other hand, too many staff changes mitigate against the comfort and serenity of profoundly handicapped people, so a very high staff ratio is needed to give adequate relief to helpers, without depriving the handicapped of the personal and individual relationships which they will develop with the team who supply daily intimate care.

CONDITIONS REQUIRING SPECIAL CARE

Multiple disability

Some mentally handicapped people have associated physical disabilities, in varying degrees. Cardiac abnormality may be present, epilepsy, mild or severe, blindness or deafness.

Specific medical treatment will be ordered for physical conditions, and nurses and helpers have the responsibility of correct administration of treatment, observation of the effect of treatment and informing prescribing physicians of any change in the condition.

Symptoms are characteristic signs of a particular state and care staff should be aware of the significance of particular symptoms.

Increasing blindness, or sudden loss of vision, irritability, sleeplessness may all point to the need for treatment and, as many profoundly disabled people have no speech, vigilant observation by nurses and care staff may be the only means of indicating that urgent attention is needed.

A group of characteristic symptoms is called a syndrome, and if this group of symptoms is peculiar to a single condition, the syndrome is specific, and may have a specific name—often associated with the original discoverer of the significance of this group of symptoms, such as Down's Syndrome.

A diagnosis may depend on the presence of all relevant symptoms, so it is important for nurses and helpers to notice any special behaviour and to note its frequency.

Epilepsy

This condition is present in a proportion of mentally handicapped people. It causes a convulsive spasm which may result in unconsciousness.

The fit may be mild, sometimes only noted by a temporary

stillness, and it may be preceded by a warning, or aura, which becomes familiar to those who care for the epileptic person, or to himself.

The person of normal intelligence, with warning of a fit, may have time to prevent himself from falling into a dangerous obstacle or fire. Mentally handicapped people are not able to help themselves and must be protected by care staff. Drugs are used to control the fits and may prevent them altogether. Special protective headgear may be worn by both children and adults to prevent head injuries caused by falling.

Sometimes a loud cry or sudden involuntary movement gives warning of a fit: the jaws are almost always tightly clenched and the tongue may be bitten or fall back and interfere with breathing.

After a fit the person may be incontinent of urine or faeces, and may fall asleep.

During a fit, helpers should prevent the person from falling or throwing his arms and legs against solid objects, or fires, and should make sure that he can breathe without obstruction and wait quietly until the fit is over before giving any further help.

Fits must always be fully reported, frequency and severity noted together with any details of special symptoms.

Autism

This condition is still not fully understood. Generally, it is a syndrome of childhood which includes profound withdrawal from people and surroundings, so that the child may appear totally unaware of the world about him.

Such children often display symptoms of great distress, terror of strange things and an insistence on activities being performed with absolute exactitude—ritual behaviour. They often make strange or bizarre movements which they perform over and over again. They may have no speech, or may only repeat meaningless phrases. Some children may also mutilate themselves.

Most mentally handicapped children do not show signs of autism, but a few may have this syndrome added to mental handicap. The condition sometimes improves after adolescence, even without special treatment. There are no specific methods of treatment, but self-mutilation must be prevented, and every attempt made by helpers and care staff to exploit physical contacts so that some communication can be made.

Behaviour which is damaging or exhausting to the child may be controlled by a corrective programme, which must be carried out immediately the behaviour begins. The technique is to *prevent* the action, not to punish it.

Severe cases of epilepsy and autism will be treated in hospital, as will some cases of severe behaviour disorder.

Each case will receive individual appropriate treatment.

LIAISON WITH FAMILY AND COMMUNITY

We have said that wherever the mentally handicapped person is living he will need some degree of care, and that in some cases this may involve special nursing skills.

Staff in subnormality hospitals may in the past have been unable to involve families in the care of mentally handicapped people because of the geographical location of the hospital and the difficulty of frequent travel. This situation is still so common that the help of family members is totally lost. But the creation of Hospital Friends Associations, now with several years of experience, has begun to bridge this gap by providing a link between family and hospital staff, which has been of real benefit to the residents in hospital.

There will however continue to be a minority of hospital residents who will have no home contacts, and as these people advance in age, so also will the age of those able to visit them and some close relatives will die, leaving them alone. There are now a number of schemes to provide a personal visitor for those who have no family. In some cases, the visitor can take the resident for outings or on holidays outside the home. The advantage to a handicapped person of an individual personal link of this sort is very great, and needs to be supported whenever possible.

SECTION SIX

Special Therapy Techniques
Physiotherapy
Water Exercises

Physical Education

Music and Eurhythmics

Movement and Drama

Play

Speech

Occupational Therapy

Drug Therapy

Behaviour Modification

Aversion Therapy

Over correction Technique

Special Therapy Techniques

There are many specialist skills which can improve the daily life of mentally handicapped people, to prevent deterioration of their condition and to enable them to benefit from teaching programmes of all kinds.

Some are designed to help them become mobile, or at least to improve their range of movement, some to deal with distressing symptoms of specific disorders—drugs may help epileptics, for example—some will help self-awareness and self-expression, through speech or movement.

There are programmes of behaviour modification which will help them in social adjustment and these specialised fields are constantly developing new and improved techniques.

Not all mentally handicapped people will need such help all the time; some may need the help of several specialist therapists at once, others may progress from one to another. Staff will need to co-operate with any specialist programme designed for people in their care, and to suggest when specialist skills may be needed.

PHYSIOTHERAPY

The advice and help of a trained physiotherapist can be vital to a handicapped infant in the early weeks of life.

As we have discussed earlier, the normal infant initiates his own movement and progresses rapidly to co-ordination of both fine and gross movements. But these natural movements have to be stimulated by others if the child is mentally handicapped, and persisted with daily if benefit is to be sustained.

The physiotherapists will observe carefully any limitations and any unnatural patterns of movement, and may use such terms as 'spastic' or 'athetoid' to describe them. Basically, spastic movements are convulsive and the affected part is constantly in uncontrollable spasm. The affected person may have spasticity of only one part of the body—one side, one limb—or all four limbs may be affected, so that they cannot work together harmoniously.

Not all spastics are mentally handicapped but when this condition is added to mental handicap it becomes a profound disability. Involuntary jerky movements of the head make speech and feeding most difficult, uncontrollable spasms of the limbs may make walking impossible. Electric or mechanical aids may be needed to use the hands and fingers, as well as for walking or guiding a wheelchair. The movements of a spastic are completely involuntary and drugs may be needed daily to ensure a degree of control.

'Flaccidity' is the opposite condition to spasticity. The muscle tone is soft and flabby, the limbs of the affected baby are rather like those of a softly-stuffed toy, and spontaneous movements are greatly reduced or absent.

Severely handicapped children have the greatest need for physiotherapy advice and the greatest need of individual care, if future crippling disablement is to be avoided. The physiotherapist will be able to design a movement treatment sequence suitable for each individual, and to show nurses, care staff and parents exactly how to carry it out. The use of lightweight plastic rollers, balls and other large light padded equipment has made it possible to carry out treatment routines in the ward, classroom or playgroup at prescribed intervals and of the correct period of time.

Treatment is aimed at correcting damaging movements and stimulating weak or indifferent natural movements, and is based upon understanding the role of normal reflexes such as gripping, rolling, crawling and the stages at which they should appear. Early training is concerned with observing the emergence of normal movement patterns and, if they are delayed, initiating movements which will stimulate them.

Older people with severe limitation of movement due to brain damage in early life cannot always be helped. In many cases they can only be given exercise and treatment to prevent the worsening of their disability. Such treatment should not be denied them, and the advice of a physiotherapist sought on an individual pattern of treatment for each person, which can be carried out by those daily concerned with their care.

Water exercises

Many movements which are difficult on land can be more effectively performed in water. In any case children, and adults, usually enjoy water play, if the temperature is agreeable and if they feel secure in the water environment.

A heated swimming bath is often accessible for mentally handicapped persons, and some pools in larger institutions even have ramps to enable people in wheelchairs to enter the water in safety and transfer to a support rail while they learn to swim.

Confidence gained in movements in water can be transferred to movements on land, and there are many other benefits for mentally handicapped children and adults.

A special method of teaching handicapped children in water was devised by two teachers at Halliwick School in North London. The principle is to make the process of learning to swim an enjoyable game, and progress is dictated by the child's own confidence in the programme. Some physiotherapists are also instructors in the Halliwick method, but all physiotherapists can advise on water exercise and how it may be beneficial in a particular case.

PHYSICAL EDUCATION

It is now generally accepted that increased mobility and the enjoyment of movement has a profound effect on the stimulation of intelligence. The immobilisation of children and adults in the old system of institutional care, where severely handicapped children were kept in cots and later in wheelchairs, not only limited their physical abilities, but denied the retarded mental development any chance of advance. Alongside individual exercise and movement the handicapped person needs also guidance to enjoy movement with others.

A remedial gymnast has been specially trained to devise patterns which will increase confidence and co-ordination of movement. Physical education is an important part of education in the special school, and nurses and care staff will need to appreciate the importance of giving support and help to severely handicapped people involved in remedial education programmes designed to help them to stand, walk and move freely.

The objective is to give the mentally handicapped person sufficient confidence to enjoy movement, and to enable him to benefit from expanding the limits of his environment and thus to continue to learn.

The handicapped child has difficulty in self-awareness, in identification of right and left, in understanding balance and co-ordination. Specially designed programmes enable him to master these skills one at a time, and eventually perhaps to work in team events.

Some children may never achieve sufficient mastery of physical skills to play games, or to take part in a team display, but even the activity of bouncing a ball, or using a low trampoline, can give pleasure and stimulation.

MUSIC AND EURHYTHMICS

Many mentally handicapped people have a well developed sense of rhythm and some are very musical, learning to play instruments of some complexity, even though severely mentally handicapped.

Music has a theraputic effect on most people, and has been used for some time in stress situations, such as a dental surgery, to induce calm. With mentally handicapped people, however, music is most valuable as a stimulant. It does not need elaborate equipment—a pleasant voice singing simple nursery rhymes to an infant can evoke responses. The ubiquitous portable radio makes instant music available almost everywhere, and one can often see groups of mentally handicapped people of all ages enjoying a pop music session and dancing in time to the music.

Music can also be used as a specially designed therapy, with movements co-ordinated to particular rhythms and melodies, setting a pattern which induces harmonious body movements. It may be possible to introduce a specially trained person to take a group of people on a regular basis, for a music and movement class. Even

EARLY HANDLING

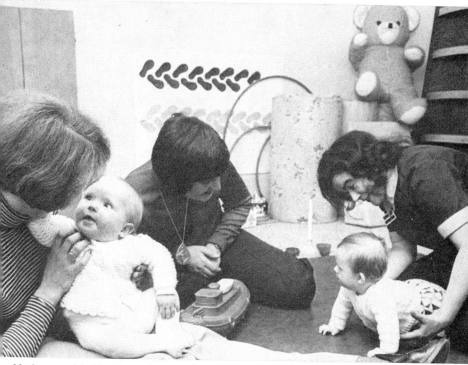

Mothers and babies learn from each other with the help of professionals.
Eye contact is an essential preliminary to communication. The mothers encourage the child to fix his gaze and contact people and objects by seeing and feeling at close quarters.

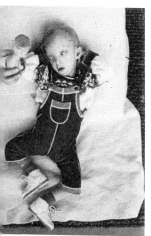 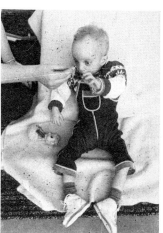 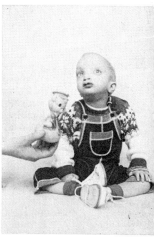

Even severely handicapped children, given stimulation and loving attention can respond and enjoy contact with others and receive pleasure from suitable toys.

STIMULATION

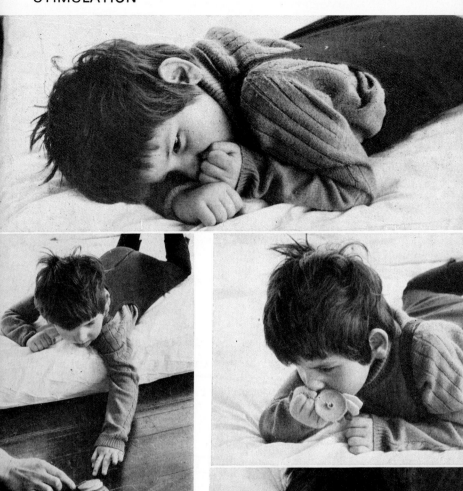

Play and stimulation is essential to children with physical and mental handicaps to prevent deterioration of muscular tone. Left alone the child would remain prone, taking little interest in his surroundings and thus becoming further deprived. Imaginative play encourages the child to reach and explore and to play happily with suitably chosen toys.

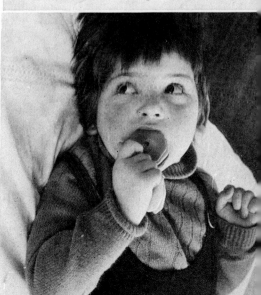

STANDING

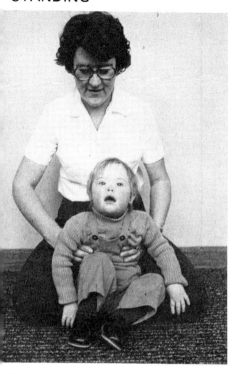 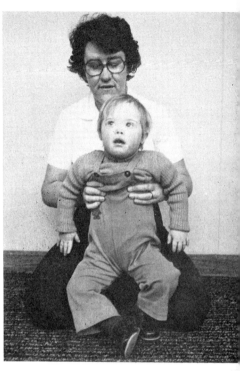

Movement is essential to increase the child's awareness and to prevent contractions. Standing is a necessary step to walking and if the child has no physical disability he can be encouraged to bear weight on his feet and gain confidence to stand alone.

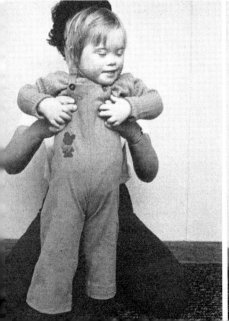 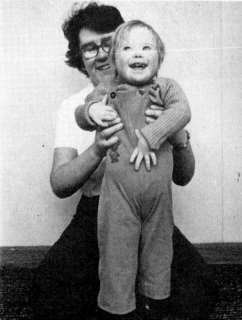

STAGES TO WALKING

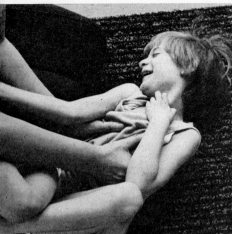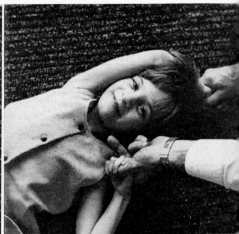

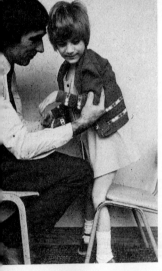

More severely physically handicapped children have a great need of mobility. Mat play, which can begin with tickling and rolling, can lead on to extension of limbs and help with a good sitting position.

Walking follows when the child has confidence in the helper and that her limitations are understood and adequate support provided.

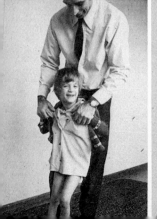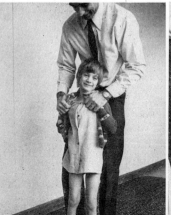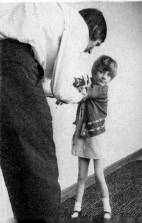

SELF-AWARENESS

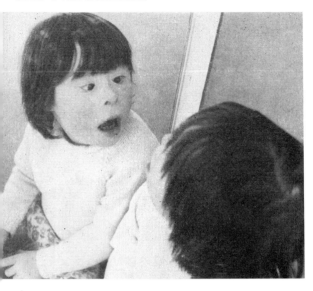

Increasing mobility allows the development of self-awareness, here shown by the use of a mirror. Many other games with fingers and toes help the child to identify himself from clothes and surroundings.

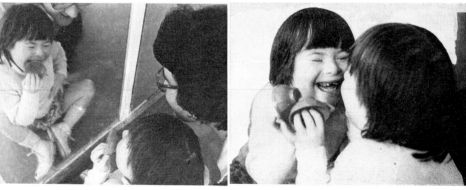

SELF-HELP

Feeding oneself is an essential life skill. The helper sits where he can see the child's face and supports the head firmly by a grasp at the angle of the jaw. His own hand grasps the spoon in the hand of the child and patterns the movement. Help is gradually withdrawn as the child learns.

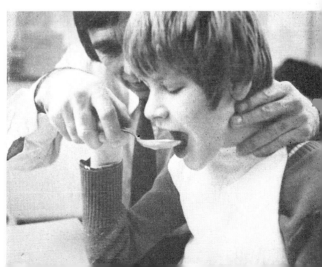

EDUCATION

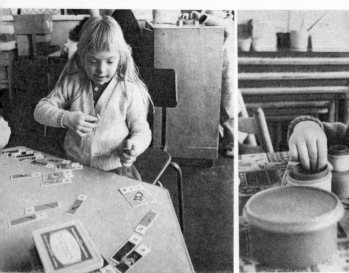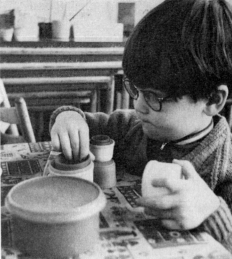

The ability to recognise symbols, match them and place them in sequence precedes reading. Children can use specially prepared material, or items from around the home to develop this ability.

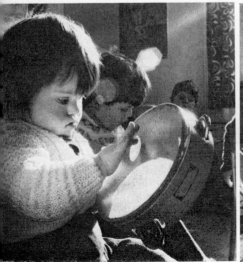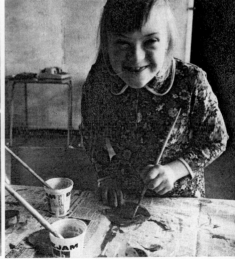

Music and painting give much pleasure and provide another means of stimulating mentally handicapped children of all ages.

LEISURE

The enjoyment of recreation is as vital to mentally handicapped people as to others. Crafts such as pottery can be learnt in groups at Adult Education Centres, reading skills acquired at school need practice to preserve and improve them.

Hobbies of woodwork and other workshop activities can be enjoyed, and painting for a hobby is always fun.

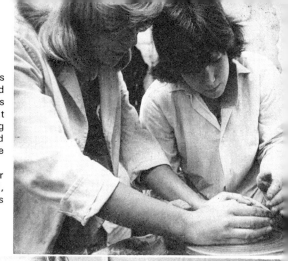

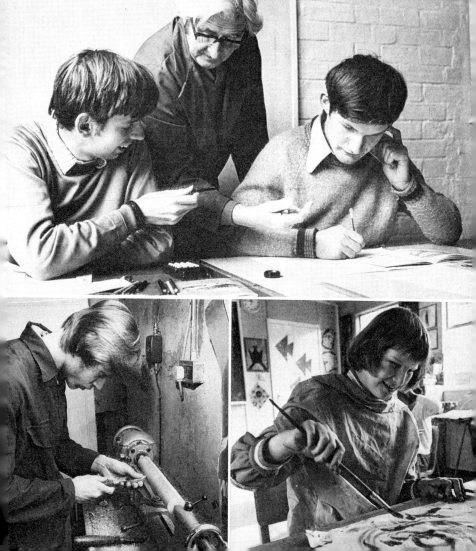

LIFE SKILLS

To live independently in the community requires mastery of some essential skills to manage money, cook and launder for oneself. With training many young adults can manage well.

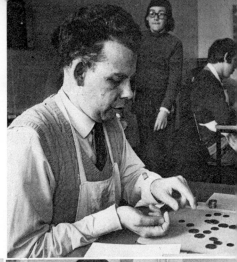

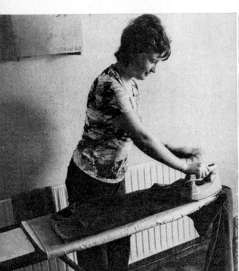

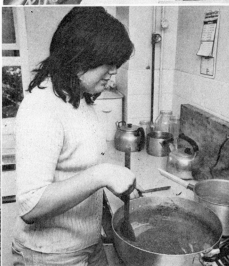

EMPLOYMENT

Some young people earn their living alongside their neighbours, in factories and farms. The personal skills of each individual are assessed and suitable work preparation courses, with appropriate supervision, ensure a better quality of life for many.

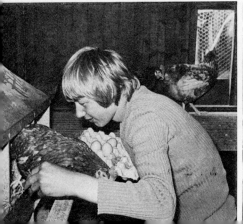

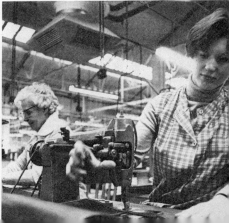

very severely retarded people can be stimulated or soothed by carefully selected music.

In a large institution, the constant use of background music at high volume, on the other hand, can be harmful, and negate the value of the planned use of music as a therapy.

All stimulating activity will increase the ability of the mentally handicapped person to learn self-help skills, and gradually to reduce dependence upon others. Nurses and care staff need to explore all possibilities for such help, and involve people from the community with special skills as part of the therapeutic team.

MOVEMENT AND DRAMA

The use of movement and drama is also now accepted to be beneficial to mentally handicapped people.

Trained tutors take small groups of handicapped people and suggest roles they may like to play in improvised situations. Commencing with very simple movements, perhaps based upon imitating the movements of birds, animals or trees, which can be observed, handicapped people, both children and adults, can become involved in group activity, dressing up and playing out again situations which they have found distressing or pleasant.

When the activity becomes part of a regular programme, the sessions will be designed to provide continuing opportunities for original ideas and individual expression.

PLAY THERAPY

Structured programmes of play are appropriate for all ages of mentally handicapped people. They are dealt with more fully in the section of the book which deals with leisure for the appropriate age group.

SPEECH THERAPY

Many mentally handicapped people have great difficulty in speaking. They often have a physical handicap—over-large tongue,

D

difficulty in swallowing and in lip movements—in addition to their slower responses which make the translation of ideas and needs into speech difficult, and listeners need much patience and time to understand what is said. It is very important to encourage any attempt at communication, so the listener should be at pains to give full attention, maintain eye-contact and if necessary repeat the phrase used until he or she fully understands what is being said. If needs are interpreted without speech, the handicapped person will eventually withdraw all effort to communicate and so lose another ability.

The speech therapist will identify the major need in each individual case. Simple swallowing exercises, blowing, chewing and other movements develop the muscles used in speech. Individual sessions devoted solely to speech improvement may need the services of the speech therapist, but this is not always possible for all those who most need help.

Speech therapy programmes have the greatest chance of success in early life, when the complex interaction between speech, language, memory and retrieval is at the vital development stage, but it is not limited to that period.

Helpers should always speak carefully to those with speech difficulty, using every opportunity to name objects and people. Even severely handicapped people can respond to a few key words, such as their own name, or a favourite toy or possession, and this small begining should be built upon and reinforced on every possible occasion. Any activity involving a quiet period on a one-to-one basis such as feeding, cutting nails, dressing, can be used to stimulate speech. The important point is to be able to convey to the handicapped person that what he wishes to communicate is as important as the patterns of speech employed by the helper.

If he reacts to pleasure or discomfort by a recognisable sound, this should be remarked upon and every time the sound is used the helper should make an appropriate response. For example, the sound indicating pleasure could be acknowledged by a smile from the helper and a carefully enunciated 'Good'. Displeasure can be marked by 'Bad' or 'No?' using not only the same word each time, but the same inflection and the same facial expression, looking directly at the person, encouraging every attempt at imitation.

For those adults with severe speech defects the mastery of a single significant word will give confidence to continue to use speech instead of signing or body movement.

For those unable to speak, there are many alternative communication systems available, and nurses and helpers will become familiar with the signs used in systems such as Paget Gorman and Makaton. One system, Blissymbolics, can be used even if the helper is quite ignorant of the system, as the handicapped person indicates on a display board or electronic indicator a desired symbol, for example, drink or lavatory, and the helper reads the word which accompanies it. Blissymbolics can be used by a person who cannot use the voice at all, and has no adequate muscle co-ordination for sign language, so it is very useful for severely retarded persons.

Whatever system is used, it is based upon the recognition by the user, the handicapped person, of the principle that one gesture or symbol has a single universal meaning which can be read or interpreted by another. It is obvious, therefore, that this gesture or symbol must be used in the same way and acknowledged in the same way each time.

If any signing or symbol system is used, all helpers and nurses must understand it, even if they are not fully proficient. The mentally handicapped person will become distressed and disturbed if he is not understood, and this point must be taken into account when any move into a different environment is contemplated, and may dictate the method of communication chosen for each individual.

Very retarded or disturbed people will often be found to have a particularly sympathetic relationship with one staff member. Whenever possible other staff members should try to acquire the key to understanding from the chosen person, rather than resort to a policy of 'Send for Nurse X, she can understand him (or manage him)'. Temperament and personality cannot be transferred, but skills, achieved by patience or intuitive understanding, can and should be transferred to others for the benefit of those in care.

Communicating with a non-verbal mentally handicapped person is a chance to learn a new language—even to design one —and brings great rewards.

OCCUPATIONAL THERAPY

Occupational therapy is not only a useful daily occupation for hands and other muscles. It aims to stimulate hand-eye co-ordination, colour discrimination and other simple skills, as well as to provide the satisfaction of a finished product : such as painting, model, basket, woven or sewn article.

For many years only very simple repetitive tasks were considered appropriate for mentally handicapped people. We now know that, like all of us, they enjoy original creative activities within their powers. By noting the activities they enjoy, programmes can be structured to develop initial skills and improve general performance. Weaving, painting, sewing, all require hand-eye co-ordination, and to complete a piece of work improves concentration and increases attention-span; while purely repetitive tasks result only in boredom and apathy.

Occupational therapists will like to hear from nursing and care staff about particular likes and potential skills, as well as about activities which need to be stimulated and encouraged.

Programmes can be designed by occupational therapists which can be carried out at other suitably equipped centres, such as a Day Training Centre, Adult Training Centre or Sheltered Workshop.

DRUG THERAPY

The modern pharmacology industry dates only from the late 1930s. Originating in Germany, it has expanded beyond imagination in the past forty years. Research and experiment daily discovers new compounds which can materially alter the physical and mental responses of the body.

Before the advent of the synthetic compounds, the only drugs available for medical treatment were those produced from natural products. It was known by the early physicians that these drugs, prepared by drying or infusing parts of plants, were themselves variable, depending upon the soil in which they were grown, and the season in which they were gathered, and that identical doses of the same product could produce vastly different effects on different people.

Today more accurate scientific methods of producing drugs for medical use can ensure that the strength and purity of each dose is of standard quality. We also have methods of measuring the exact response of any individual to a prescribed dosage. What we still *cannot* do is to predict exactly how the working of a prescribed drug will be affected by changes in the health and mental balance of a person. Even changes in his way of life, or simple changes or additions to his diet, may alter a person's reactions to a drug. People have markedly individual responses even to common foods such as milk, cheese, shellfish, alcohol; and their physical health and state of mind may dramatically alter from time to time even these individual responses to diet.

Thus when a drug is prescribed for a mentally handicapped person, no less than for the rest of us, we need to know why it is being prescribed, how long we should continue to use it, and what the effects may be.

Any new drug must be administered with care and the effect observed and monitored. The dose may need minute adjustment to suit the individual : it should relieve his distress, but not superimpose a second condition to aggravate the first. All drugs must be kept in locked and secure cupboards or stores.

People who are mentally handicapped may be said to live in a state of 'altered awareness' : their consciousness is different from what we understand as the norm. The difference may be so slight as to pass almost unnoticed : the person may just seem to be slow. Or it may be profoundly different, and be expressed in bizarre and violently disturbed behaviour, which may exhaust and distress both the person affected and those around him. These episodes may not last long, and new drugs have made it possible to control them, and obviate the need for the old practices of physical restraint and custody designed to prevent them injuring themselves or others.

There are many hundreds of compounds currently available to help in achieving a balance of mind which will enable a person to function without undue stress.

Drugs fall into five commonly accepted groups, according to the effect they produce.

(1) The Tranquillisers. Given to provide relief from any form of stress which is temporarily damaging. Most people today have been prescribed tranquillisers at some time or other, usually for a brief period in their lives when they were under exceptional strain. Some of the well known travel sickness pills come into this category. Their function is to remove anxiety, while at the same time enabling the person to continue (within certain limits) his normal activities.

(2) Sedatives. These are sleeping pills, which, once again, are in common use today by many people who, because of temporary mental or physical distress, cannot sleep or rest sufficiently to function normally.

(3) The Hypnotics. These are much more powerful drugs, which are available for more distressing states of restlessness and sleeplessness. Some can also be prescribed for convulsions and epilepsy.

(4) Anti-depressants. As the name implies, these drugs relieve symptoms of anxiety and depression. Such symptoms may include those of a physical illness without apparent physical cause, called psychosomatic illness.

(5) Psycho-stimulants. These drugs are available for people who have withdrawn totally from their surroundings and present the appearance of being in another world—sometimes even comatose. Their action is to intensify stimulation.

All these drugs are available for use, but their abuse is a very real danger.

All are substances foreign to the human body, and all must be eliminated from it by the normal processes of the liver, kidneys and lungs. How efficiently these organs perform, differs in each individual; and no drug can be given day in, day out, without some adverse effects.

Mentally handicapped people cannot appreciate for themselves the dangers implicit in drug administration or in the effect of missing a needed dose, so a system of very accurate recording by those who live with and help them is essential. Changes in the reaction to the drug need to be reported at once to the prescribing doctor; and if the person becomes physically ill, from any common cause such as a cold, accident or infectious disease, information about the drug and the usual response to it may be vital to the good conduct of his illness.

It is impossible for anyone to be knowledgeable about every drug in common daily use. What it is essential for those responsible for mentally handicapped people to know, is :

(1) Why the drug is prescribed;
(2) Details of the method of administration—how often, for how long;
(3) To whom any adverse reactions should be immediately reported;
(4) The importance of security in the storage of any potent drug—it should be locked away from children and others who might take it irresponsibly;
(5) How to record the date, time and amount of all prescribed drugs given.

BEHAVIOUR MODIFICATION

This is a comparatively new technique. It has been used to change political attitudes in times of conflict to condition susceptible people to alter their convictions and outlook and its therapeutic use was considered warily for some time.

Behaviour can be modified by a system involving punishment or reward, or a combination of both. Behaviour modification thus has some of the elements of ordinary training methods, but differs in that it is not always based upon the desire or wishes of the person concerned and may, in fact, be actively resisted by him. It thus raises moral questions some of which are still unresolved.

In simple terms, we are all conditioned from infancy to modify our behaviour, and as young children we frequently resented and resisted it. Who has not seen a red-faced screaming child being dragged through some social situation which he is not old enough to accept as reasonable?

With mentally handicapped persons, behaviour modification may be used to change patterns of individual behaviour which cause annoyance to others, or even cause others to reject the person. Regurgitating food, faecal incontinence and constant public masturbation are possible examples. All give pleasurable sensations, which in the life of the very profoundly retarded may be rare, but they also further cut that person off from others.

Behaviour is modified by individual programmes incorporating reward for the desired behaviour, and sometimes punishment for undesirable behaviour. Rewards can be simple approval—'Good girl', a smile, a hug, or a chance to hear a loved piece of music, or a treat such as an outing or specially liked food. Punishment can be simply the withdrawal of approval, or removal for short periods from the group. It is never physical punishment.

The programme must be absolutely consistent, the desired result must always be rewarded in the same way, and it must be persisted in until the modified behaviour becomes automatic.

Punishing mentally handicapped persons by shouting or hitting them is not only cruel, it is useless. The only effect is so to confuse them that they are unable to understand what they are supposed to be doing, or to remember what they have previously learned.

It requires endless patience and total tenacity to persevere with any behaviour modification programme which involves a major change of conduct. Unless this commitment is present it is unlikely that there will be any success, and the behaviour of the handicapped person may actually grow worse as a result of a failed programme.

To have any chance of an improved result the programme must

have a limited aim : one step at a time must be the rule, each small success leading to another. Expert help from an educational psychologist may help to define the best approach for each person.

Observation over a sufficient period will show under what circumstances the undesirable behaviour happens most often : what triggers off a bout of head-banging, for example. Sometimes removal of the cause alone will effect a change in the behaviour, lessening the frequency and hopefully replacing it with a less damaging response.

More observation will reveal the likes and dislikes of each person, that is identify what can best be used to reward or punish. Punishment—a sharp 'No', removal from the group—must be immediate so that it is clearly connected with the behaviour in the mind of the person being admonished, and it must never be prolonged. To remove a child from the group for a few minutes is sufficient; to keep him away longer only enables him to forget what he was removed for. Deep seated fears, such as fears of the dark or of water, must never be exploited in punishment : terror and confusion can only worsen his behaviour and adversely affect future programmes.

Used with skill and extreme selectivity, only for behaviour which is against the best interest of the mentally handicapped person, modification therapy is a useful tool. But it can be a dangerous method in the hands of unskilled persons who may use it to correct behaviour which in their view is undesirable, but which in reality is protective to the individual, and its removal may result in a new, and even less desirable pattern.

More usually behaviour modification is part of a planned training programme, such as is needed by mentally handicapped adults leaving school or home or hospital to live in the community. To some extent such people have established behaviour adapted to supervision by others—they wait to be told what to do in their daily lives. So in addition to learning simple life skills, they have also to adopt a more independent pattern of general behaviour and this can be achieved by gradually introduced modification programme.

AVERSION THERAPY

An extreme method of behaviour modification is Aversion Therapy. This method is used to eliminate behaviour which is held to be extremely damaging either to the subject or to others, and works by giving an unpleasant shock each time the undesirable behaviour is seen. It has been used with the consent of the addicted person to deal with alcoholism, drug abuse and some criminal activities.

In the case of mentally handicapped persons, aversion therapy has been used when all else has failed to cure extreme self-mutilating behaviour. Some severely handicapped children, and a few adults, bite and scratch their own bodies, bang their heads against hard surfaces, gouge their eyes and even threaten their own lives. It is thought that in such cases the degree of mental damage is so profound, and the messages reaching the brain cells in such confusion, that only the sensation of pain, summoned at will, is meaningful to the afflicted person.

Methods of distraction and a degree of restraint will be tried first, and only when all other methods have failed will some practitioners advise aversion therapy.

OVER-CORRECTION TECHNIQUE

This is method of dealing with behaviour which is damaging to a child or adult, even if not so severely damaging as to be life-threatening.

The technique is planned after a careful assessment and evaluation of the degree and frequency of the damaging behaviour.

The most commonly observed patterns of such behaviour are constant body rocking, head banging or picking and plucking at the skin. This often absorbs the energies of the person to such a degree that he cannot be distracted from it to more rewarding activities, so it is very destructive to learning. Teachers in a special school may indeed conclude, if the problem is very severe, that such a child cannot be educated in a class group. If he is not to lose the benefit of social interaction with other children, the behaviour must be eradicated.

The method involves a set of formal corrective movements designed to employ the hands and arms in another activity in such a way as to preclude the destructive behaviour. For example, if the child starts a body rocking movement, or head banging, the teacher or helper immediately stands behind the child, and taking one hand in each of his own, goes through a specially devised routine. This may involve, for instance, fully extending the arms to the side of the body and above the head, crossing the arms over at waist level, and so on. The helper will continue this exercise for a minute or more—the exact time will be specified by the psychologist designing the programme.

The routine is then carried out on every occasion the destructive behaviour is seen, and repeated until the intervals between the destructive bouts lessen to a tolerable level.

There have been some recorded studies on the effect of this form of therapy, and it will no doubt be further developed and explored.

Staff or helper ratios will dictate the conditions under which it can be used.

SECTION SEVEN

Mentally Handicapped People in the Community

Mentally Handicapped People in the Community

All that has been described in general terms in the first six sections of this book applies to mentally handicapped people, both children and adults, whether they live in institutions or in homes in the community.

Their needs, and programmes designed to supply these needs, will be carried out by those who are at hand to help them. These needs will change as they pass from infancy into childhood and from school days to adult life.

Each country will make such provision for support to families as is deemed appropriate and which is in line with social and economic attitudes of that country.

We have taken the United Kingdom provisions as a model for this book, but many of the principles are now accepted internationally. The International League of Societies for the Mentally Handicapped, an association of voluntary bodies, with over 80 member societies all over the world defined the Rights of Mentally Handicapped Persons at an international assembly in Jerusalem in 1968.

This Declaration, adopted in 1971 by the General Assembly of the United Nations forms the framework within which all members of the United Nations work today. These Rights are :

Declaration of general and special rights of the mentally retarded

Whereas the universal declaration of human rights, adopted by the United Nations, proclaims that all of the human family, without distinction of any kind, have equal and inalienable rights of human dignity and freedom;

Whereas the declaration of the rights of the child, adopted by the United Nations, proclaims the rights of the physically, mentally or socially handicapped child to special treatment, education and care required by his particular condition.

Now Therefore

The International League of Societies for the Mentally Handicapped expresses the general and special rights of the mentally retarded as follows :

ARTICLE I

The mentally retarded person has the same basic rights as other citizens of the same country and same age.

ARTICLE II

The mentally retarded person has a right to proper medical care and physical restoration and to such education, training, habilitation and guidance as will enable him to develop his ability and potential to the fullest possible extent, no matter how severe his degree of disability. No mentally handicapped person should be deprived of such services by reason of the costs involved.

ARTICLE III

The mentally retarded person has a right to economic security and to a decent standard of living. He has a right to productive work or to other meaningful occupation.

ARTICLE IV

The mentally retarded person has a right to live with his own family or with fosterparents; to participate in all aspects of community life, and to be provided with appropriate leisure time activities. If care in an institution becomes necessary it should be in surroundings and under circumstances as close to normal living as possible.

ARTICLE V

The mentally retarded person has a right to a qualified guardian when this is required to protect his personal wellbeing and interest. No person rendering direct services to the mentally retarded should also serve as his guardian.

ARTICLE VI

The mentally retarded person has a right to protection from exploitation, abuse and degrading treatment. If accused, he has a right to a fair trial with full recognition being given to his degree of responsibility.

ARTICLE VII

Some mentally retarded persons may be unable, due to the severity of their handicap, to exercise for themselves all of their rights in a meaningful way. For others, modification of some sort or all of these rights is appropriate. The procedure used for modification or denial of rights must contain proper legal safeguards against every form of abuse, must be based on an evaluation of the social capability of the mentally retarded person by qualified experts and must be subject to periodic reviews and to the right of appeal to higher authorities.

ABOVE ALL

THE MENTALLY RETARDED PERSON

HAS THE RIGHT TO RESPECT.

October 24, 1968.

It will be seen that there is a recognition of general rights as citizens, and a recognition of special needs throughout life.

We need to be aware of these special needs at different ages, and how the support required can be supplied by community resources.

For easy reference, the conditions relevant to the various stages of development are divided into sections, with the community support services generally available described so that staff who are working with families will be aware of facilities which support the parents, and staff responsible for residential care may select the information appropriate to the age group for whom they care.

CREATING A DOMESTIC ENVIRONMENT

To provide a homely and familiar place for mentally handicapped people presents a problem no different in kind from providing it for others, but it is different in degree, because it is much more difficult to find out from mentally handicapped people themselves what they find homely and comforting.

If we can put ourselves in the position of having to make a new home in a new country, where climate, rules and household utensils are all quite different from those in our familiar homes, we may have some idea of what is involved.

First, we should all wish to take with us something from our old home, especially those things we feel to be essential to us. What is essential will vary according to individuals. Some cannot live without books, others want musical records or an instrument they like to play, pictures, flowers and plants, or pet animals. We also all require our own personal equipment: clothing, shoes, toilet articles, towels and some special items of linen.

If you can think what you would need in these circumstances, you may be able to analyse why some are so important, and others less so, and so help the handicapped people to make their own choices.

Preparing for change

Mentally handicapped children leaving one home for another residential placement suffer a severely traumatic experience. Whatever we may do, the new environment cannot exactly match the old one.

Even if we can arrange for parents to accompany the child,

and stay for a few days—and this is by no means a common arrangement—the child must adapt himself to new people as best he can. He has also to adapt to a new daily routine, and to new furnishings, new equipment and new personal items.

To leave as many familiar things with him as possible will lessen the violent effects of the change and protect him a little from the need to make a total adaptation at once. His own clothing, a familiar toy or other loved object, will make the surroundings less strange.

To help adults to adjust to change requires the same sensitivity, the same ability to put oneself into the position of the other, and so help the mentally handicapped person through a difficult period. He probably cannot put into words the fears and anxieties he feels, and may be able to demonstrate it only by bizzare and difficult behaviour.

Elderly people, and those who have been ill for some time in an institution, find that the return to their own home brings an immediate feeling of comfort. The familiar is therapeutic, the converse is equally true : in a state of illness or distress, a strange and threatening environment may increase the severity of the symptoms.

With this in mind, all care staff receiving new residents, children or adults, should do everything possible to minimise the strange and new environment.

Homeliness will relate also to what has been experienced as 'home'—a child arriving for a boarding school place who has had no other children around him at home will need help to adapt to the greater numbers, more noise and more activity than he is used to. A child from a large family may feel lost and lonely if he is suddenly removed to a small unit. The same is true for adults. Transitions must be planned to give a gradual adjustment to new circumstances.

Making a home
What then makes a 'home' of a new 'living place'? Certainly, it requires the opportunity to express one's personal tastes in one's environment—favourite colours and furnishings, pictures and

photographs, all promote a feeling of belonging, so that each individual identifies with that house, that room, that bed.

The companionship of others of like interest also helps, as well as privacy when it is wanted, and freedom to come and go and to have some power over one's immediate environment, to choose a picture or bedcover for oneself.

Mentally handicapped people cannot always express their needs or their feelings, but this does not mean that they have none, or that they are perfectly content to accept those of others.

A homely environment is not created by furnishings and personal belongings only, but by the feeling of being a part of a small, warm and caring unit, among people who understand your needs and will compromise when your needs conflict with theirs, and where you can relax and be yourself.

Any shared living environment presents problems of adapting to other residents, of sharing household chores equitably, of taking responsibility for not inflicting your own unsocial behaviour on your companions.

Mentally handicapped people need a good deal of support and guidance during this period of adjustment, and creating the right atmosphere of acceptance and trust will give confidence and enable new residents to settle in well.

A good home is one where not only the family, but all who come as visitors feel at home. The welcome given to others reflects the balance and acceptance of others which already exists within.

No amount of careful design, personal clothing and high standard of maintenance can create a homely environment. This comes from care and concern and the ability to ask oneself 'would I like to live here?' If the answer to that question is not a clear 'yes', it is time to analyse what is wrong, and to make some definite attempts to put things right.

Too many rigid rules, incompatible residents, too much emphasis on tidiness and order, or too little, the absence of familiar objects or pets, residences designed to standards which are unfamiliar, either too far above or below what has been earlier experienced, will all cause unnecessary distress.

If the residents are involved to the maximum degree possible in the planning and design of the units in which they are to live, and encouraged to participate in the daily management of their lives, such units will become 'home'.

Staff changes also threaten the security of a home, though some can be tolerated if there is always at least a firm core of permanent staff. This, too, is easiest to achieve if the conditions are 'homely' for the staff as well as for those for whom they care.

Elaborately purpose-built units, furnished to a common high standard by remote administrative systems, may create hotels, but never homes. When new units are planned, those who are to live in them and those who will work in them have a contribution to make, which is even more important if the residence is likely to be home for some considerable time.

Such units are nowadays ordinary houses on ordinary estates, among other tenants or house owners. The mentally handicapped residents and their helpers will have the best chance of acceptance if their home is as reasonably like those of their neighbours as possible, both outwardly and in its furnishings, particularly those which can be seen by the neighbours: fresh curtains, clean windows, neat front doors and gardens.

But caring for the home in which they live needs also to be taught. One experimental unsupported group home became conspicuous when the mentally handicapped residents innocently extended their wallpapering activities to the front door, making it both personal and homely in their own eyes, but less so to their neighbours'. Managing a home, keeping it tidy, attending to the garden, doing the washing, having respect for one's neighbours by avoiding very noisy music from radio or records, is often not well done by ordinary people, but they may escape unchallenged because they have already been accepted. Much of what newly arrived mentally handicapped residents do is subject to much more severe scrutiny, and for this reason, if no other, helpers and care assistants need to give extra vigilance in teaching and supervising social behaviour in the home situation.

Wherever mentally handicapped people live, some support services are essential. These will vary in degree, relative to the degree of handicap. Some people require only the very minimum of supervision, of the type given by a warden of a group of residences for elderly people; others need daily assistance with the basic tasks of living.

At this time there is very great disparity in the services provided, in quality, type and quantity, from one area of the country to another.

HOME AND FAMILY SUPPORT SERVICES

The family doctor and health visitor provide health care for everyone, handicapped or not, and the service they offer is statutory. As the numbers of mentally handicapped people in any one residential area may be small, however, these people may not have specialised knowledge of mental handicap.

The vital few weeks after the mother returns from hospital with a new baby who is mentally handicapped are at present covered by the health visitor. But some areas also have a special liaison system between the hospital where the baby was born and the community service, and provide a specially trained community nurse to support the family at this time. In other areas the follow-up from the maternity hospital to the community support services is less good and the parents may be left without advice and help.

Mentally handicapped babies have greater difficulty in adjustment to change than other babies, and problems of feeding, sleep and infections, particularly upper respiratory infections, are common.

The years from birth to two years are so important that every available source of help must be explored, for the baby needs special education techniques even at this early age. It should be remembered that the Social Services do not automatically receive notice of the arrival of a mentally handicapped baby, so the parents will need to inform the local office that they may require help. At the regular baby clinic all mothers can be advised by the nurses and the doctor in attendance, but some mothers are so distressed by their baby's handicap that they do not even attend the clinic. Yet in these early weeks much may be happening which is vitally important to the future welfare of the child, and all available resources should be mobilised to help the family, for the health and well-being of the family will always contribute the major part of any future influences on the handicapped person. Time and skill expended on counselling advice, and the transfer of skills to the parents, become more important at this time than any other.

Voluntary agencies

A great deal of help can be given by voluntary agencies at this time. Not all parents wish to contact other parents with similar problems, but it is important that the family make a link with someone they can trust and whose help they will call upon. Withdrawal into a closed world denies the child the help he will need. Family circumstances vary so much, and the personalities of parents, that no one agency will be acceptable to all. Many voluntary agencies offer a variety of services, provided by other parents of handicapped babies and by professional staff.

Early education provisions

After two years of age the local authority should make provision for any child in need of special education by reasons of disability. Nursery classes and play groups now exist in most areas, where mentally handicapped infants can join other small children in the group. The argument for this integration is that if mentally handicapped children can play and learn alongside children without handicap at this age, they see daily a model of normal behaviour to imitate, rather than remain 'stuck' in a retarded state. There are disadvantages however if the group is too large, is housed in unsatisfactory conditions or is too far from the child's home. A small group of children with a sufficient number of staff gives the best results, as individual attention is needed for the handicapped infant.

At five years, or earlier in some cases, the child will enter the education system proper. Every child is legally entitled to education appropriate to his needs (Education Act 1971). Very severely retarded children may need to be in a residential school, either on a weekly boarding basis, or, if such a school is not available locally, throughout the term.

THE CHILD AT HOME

Less severely handicapped children may attend an ESN(M) day school in the local area.

Schools will have a staff of teachers, care assistants and trained nurses and maintain strong links with families whenever possible.

The school nurse observes the children daily for signs of illness or infection, attends to first aid and removal to hospital should treatment be needed, and supervises the administration of medicines. She will also note any signs that the child cannot see or hear normally, needs physiotherapy or other help.

During the school life of the child, usually up to 16 years, the umbrella of the school health service will cover all his health and dental care.

The family can approach the Social Services for assistance with holidays, transport and special appliances, including adaptations to the home, required for example if the child has to use a wheelchair or walking frame, or is incontinent. The range of statutory benefits available is constantly changing, and eligibility for each is often determined on an individual basis, so the task of making sure that every family has all benefits to which it is entitled may involve some persistence. There is in addition often insufficient co-operation between school, doctor and social services, though the development of community mental handicap teams may help to improve this.

Most mentally handicapped children of school age live with their families for most of the year; though in some schools, programmes continue through the periods of school holidays, there are always times when the family needs respite periods.

Holidays, with the handicapped child, or without, are essential to the well-being of those who care for him, and there are many schemes available. Financial help for such holidays is sometimes available from local authorities.

Leisure facilities specially designed for mentally handicapped people are provided for by some voluntary agencies. The National Federation of Gateway Clubs has a club in almost every area, and Riding for the Disabled gives help to those who can enjoy this activity.

RESIDENTIAL HOMES

If the child is deprived, for any reason, of family life, he may live in a residential home provided by the Social Services Department of the local authority, or by a voluntary agency. The home tries to meet the primary need of any child for love, care and individual attention, and the staff are, in effect, acting as parents. Not many of them however see the task as a life-long commitment, so the major problem is rapid staff turn-over in establishments. If there is some degree of permanence in the senior staff appointments so that there is some stability and continuance of daily routine, it is possible that the damaging effect of this turn-over may be lessened. Change and upheavals have a traumatic effect on the young child and this is especially marked if the child is handicapped. He becomes bewildered and disorientated and may revert to patterns of behaviour appropriate to a much younger child.

Children who have been bereaved by the death of a parent, or who have suffered from other breadowns in family life, require special help in adapting to a new home, and time to make a close bond with another adult. If they have to share this response between several different members of staff their distress increases and they may completely withdraw.

Small units of fewer than ten places can provide the best environment for children and adults alike, and if these are located in ordinary houses in a residential area they have the added advantage that, like ordinary families, the residents can live within the same home for as long as they need.

Staff of units providing care and supervision may be housed in the same building, like parents, or close at hand in adjoining units, but they must always provide close, continuing care for the children.

HOSTELS AND GROUP HOMES

Many ordinary children leave home after the school years, and provision for mentally handicapped young people to live away from home is made in several ways. Hostels vary in size, from those with under eight places to some with over forty. Obviously, a hostel of forty cannot be a home, and the management of a unit of this size takes on an institutional character.

A small hostel may be supervised by one warden, with services provided for domestic cleaning and maintenance. The most successful schemes have been those which mix residents of different ability and sex in small units, so that each can contribute to the other. Some residents may be in open employment, some in sheltered workshops or Adult Training Centres, and some may remain in the home or hostel during the day, providing meals and doing the laundry and other chores on behalf of the family group.

Very careful preparation for independent living is the key to success, together with unobtrusive but vigilant supervision in the early stages. Some experiments in group homes fail because this need for continuing care has not been realised. It may take more than a year for a pattern of family life to be established. A group of mentally handicapped people will be exposed to the same stresses and strains as any other family : they will have emotional upsets, become ill, lose jobs, encounter unexpected difficulties, and until they have had the opportunity to acquire, through experience, the skill to deal with their problems they will need caring, professional support.

Staff are constantly in a vulnerable position. If they do not take sufficient care they are accused of negligence, if they take too much, of authoritarian interference. They share this dilemma with all parents, but whereas the parent is unanswerable, in most cases, only to himself, professional staff are answerable to the community.

A recent judgement on personal liability may provide a guide line.

The parents of a child who had injured another, unintentionally in play, were sued by the injured child's parents on the grounds that they were responsible for the actions of the child. The Court's judgement stated that no one can be held liable for the actions of another person, only for his own; but that if the parents had not instructed the child in terms acceptable to his intelligence of the dangers inherent in the toy, they would be liable. The parents successfully proved that they had given adequate instruction.

It would seem, therefore, that those staff responsible, by virtue of their conditions of employment, for ensuring that mentally handicapped people are not a danger to themselves or others, discharge their responsibility by giving adequate instruction and supervision *related to the ability of the handicapped person.* To decide how much instruction and supervision is needed demands careful observation, knowledge of the background of the handicapped person and knowledge of appropriate teaching and educational techniques.

Selection of people to live in group homes or hostels may need a team of those who have specialist knowledge, but if the special needs of each resident are fully understood and provided for, hopes for success may be well fulfilled. Haphazard grouping, on the other hand, without full information or adequate support, is bound to result in disaster, and may so damage the community response to one hostel or group home as to preclude the setting up others in the same locality.

MIXED ABILITY HOUSING

There have been pilot schemes where adult students at centres of higher education or working people share living accommodation with mentally handicapped people. The advantages would appear to be that the residents of above average ability can assist in the decision-making functions and the lower ability group carry out communal tasks which do not require the higher intelligence skills. Some extensions of the concept are planned and should be watched with interest.

Though of course such a scheme could deteriorate into a 'slave and master' situation, if there is a common acceptance of the value of different skills, and of the importance of understanding people of all levels of ability, it could provide another pattern of residence within the community, outside the institution. The inherent lack of permanence in such a project, however, makes it more suitable as a transition scheme than a settled solution, unless the administration of the residence is vested in some continuing body.

INDIVIDUAL HOUSING

Some mentally handicapped people marry and live as couples in ordinary flats and houses. If a mentally handicapped person marries a normal partner, the problem is usually well contained by the support of the partner and the families concerned. But if both are mentally handicapped, standards of housekeeping may be low and, in some cases, actually present a health or safety hazard. Staff providing support for less able people need to be alert for signs of potential hazards and devise simple, easily understood procedures to help. The use of fire guards, protection of electrical appliances and cooking stoves, are obvious safety measures. But utensils left on stairs, rubbish not properly dealt with and food left uncovered and available for contamination are less obvious perils, though equally dangerous. The home is a dangerous environment for intelligent people—more accidents occur there than in traffic—and help is certainly needed by mentally handicapped people to avoid them.

'Help' is the operative word—mentally handicapped adults, no less than others, need to be encouraged to define their own needs and devise methods of coping with them, not to have their lives taken over by others. The problem lies in their limited ability to predict the consequences of actions and to plan a new sequence for themselves. They can remember and act upon past experience, but not anticipate new events. Thus it is important to visit regularly, to request help from neighbours, who can give very real support if sympathetically approached, and to be alert to any changes in the living conditions of mentally handicapped people which may need immediate intervention.

VILLAGE COMMUNITIES

There are a number of voluntary organisations which run village communities for mentally handicapped persons. The life of both staff and residents is largely catered for within the boundaries of the community. All live within its confines, though some may go outside daily, for school or other activity. Other villages are almost totally self-supporting, providing education, growing food, baking bread, cultivating the land and maintaining the properties and equipment within it.

There are long waiting lists for many village communities, and for most there is a selection on entry which is based upon the contribution that the individual can make. Villages based upon a rural or craft model will take people with sufficient physical or manual skill to be capable of instruction and of effective work. Others ask only that those coming to live are socially co-operative. The Rudolf Steiner schools offer a community life throughout the school years, together with a therapeutic education. Fees for the children are paid by the parents or by means of grants from local authorities. Staff receive no salaries, but share in all activities of the community and all their needs are met.

There are also village communities for adults set up on Steiner principles. The criteria for admission are that the handicapped adult should wish to live in the community, and be temperamentally able to benefit from it.

It is calculated that about 20 percent of all mentally handicapped school leavers will not be able to function without supervision in community life—largely because of their inability to cope with the complexity of salaries and contributions to pensions and other benefits, or to organise their spending to take account of daily needs. Within the village community they are spared such concern, contributing their labour and skills to a common pool, from which all their practical needs are met. The basic need for satisfaction in work and of producing goods and services needed by others is itself often a character developing activity and an enrichment of life; for the mentally handicapped person, no less than others, needs to feel that he is valuable and that his life has function and purpose.

FLEXIBILITY OF PROVISIONS

It will be seen that the key to satisfactory intergration of the mentally handicapped people in any community is the provision of amenities which can be changed or adapted for particular needs. The huge subnormality hospital is thus a problem simply because to change its essential structure is well-nigh impossible, no matter how much is expended.

To build purpose-designed units may be equally short-sighted, if they are not capable of subsequent adaptation to future needs. Technological advances bring each year aids and systems undreamt of earlier, which make some of our current amenities out of date even as they are being built. Small pilot projects at least give the chance of experimentation without colossal expense.

The old idea that big is beautiful and bigger is better, is being challenged. The huge new acute hospitals, built to centralise expensive services and equipment, are proving vulnerable to breakdown by human and mechanical failures which make them more dangerous by virtue of their very size. New private hospitals are returning to the older cottage hospital model in respect of size at least.

Even methods of providing essential services, especially of heating, are currently under intense scrutiny. New forms of energy utilisation will drastically affect the design of new buildings and compel modifications to existing ones.

Provisions for mentally handicapped people living in the community must be planned to take into account the changing patterns of daily life.

SECTION EIGHT

The new-born and infant

Telling the Parents

First steps

Handling the baby

Feeding

Weaning

Sleeping

Fresh Air

Improving muscle tone

Sitting

The two-year-old and toddler

Play group

Common infections

Incubation chart

Immunisation chart

Symptoms of Common Fevers

Measles, German measles (Rubella)

Mumps, Chicken pox

Whooping Cough, Diphtheria

The new-born and infant

Every child born is part of a family, and if he is the first child, completes the family and initiates the role of husband and wife as parents. His family, his parents, are crucial to his development and no discussion on the needs of the newly born can ignore the aspects of parental involvement.

It is now fully accepted that the bond between mother and baby is forged in the first few hours—even moments—after birth, and that delay in this initial bond may materially affect the future relationship. The mother wants immediately to hold her child, to fondle and examine him, and the child needs this intimate contact. So if a child is born with some recognisable physical defect—is slow to breathe, or needs other medical care—and the moment when he and the mother meet for the first time is delayed, the response of each may be adversely affected. Medical staff need to be sensitive to this, and to ensure that any delay is as short as possible.

If the child is handicapped the responsibility of giving the information to the new parents, too, is likely to be that of a member of the medical staff. This task is indeed an awesome one. The most common reaction to such news is an intolerable sense of grief and loss, equal to news of a breavement, so he who carries the news becomes associated with this anguish. But in that first discovery of the handicap, the pattern of the whole future relationships in the family may be set, so the situation calls for very great sensitivity and awareness.

From a background of wide experience, the most commonly advise procedure is for the news not to be delayed unduly; but if the disability is not immediately apparent, the mother and baby should not be denied the initial close encounter simply to provide time for detailed clinical assessment. Love first, science later should be the rule.

E

When examination has confirmed that there is definite evidence of mental handicap, both parents should be told together, in conditions of reasonable privacy and comfort, given the opportunity to ask some questions, then left to comfort and support each other. The baby is thus seen as one unit of a family, his eventual happiness and care depending upon his family's strength and support.

Nursing staff in general maternity units may not see many mentally handicapped babies; but it may help them to understand that the mother whose baby is born handicapped undergoes a traumatic experience, no less than the mother whose baby is still-born. In some ways her plight is worse, for there is no finality in her sorrow, only a continuing anxiety and alarm.

Both parents may need skilled counselling and both will need extra care. The family doctor should be informed *at once* so that he may be alert to the needs of the father returning home alone to face a problem of which in many cases he knows nothing.

Marriage breakdowns in parents of handicapped children is not rare, and often it is the father who leaves the wife and child. No effort should be spared by staff to include the father in the caring—his reactions may not be so evident as those of the mother, but they may run none the less deep for that. He, too, looked forward to the birth of the child, made plans for the future, and was proud that he would have a place in the continuance of human life.

TELLING THE PARENTS

It is tremendously important that all those in contact with the family speak with the same voice. This requires a definite policy on the part of all those concerned as to *who* says what, *what* is said, and when.

If there are students and care assistants, they need to know what they should say, and what kind of questions need to be referred to a senior staff member. Half-understood statements retailed to parents can cause great damage and be very difficult to eradicate.

Most parents will prefer a diagnosis—in terms which they themselves can use in informing the rest of their family and friends. Thus clinical terms may not be appropriate. Some parents may not fully understand medical terms or wish to repeat them. It may be enough to say that the baby has a handicap, and that the degree of handicap and its effect cannot be known precisely. Other parents may fully understand what is meant by 'Down's Syndrome' for example. Consultants and senior staff should give some guidance to care staff as to the terms to use in particular cases.

Certainly, only the information which is useful should be given to parents, and staff should not be afraid to say 'we don't know', if they honestly do not know. They should, however, be informed upon the questions which are most likely to be asked.

The first one is usually Why?—Why did it happen and why to me?

Often, to this question, there is no exact answer, and the best help to the parents is to help them to see that the answer to Why? is less important at this very early stage than 'What can I do?'

There is a very great deal which can be done and *must* be done to take maximum advantage of the learning ability of the very young infant. The mother needs to be immediately involved, and the father shown how he can help, not only by supporting the mother but by actively participating in his baby's care and progress.

FIRST STEPS

Communication must be established between mother and baby as soon after birth as possible. Initially, this is achieved by eye contact, by gazing at the child and encouraging the baby to fix his gaze back on the face of the mother.

The little drawings on page 132 show vividly the great importance of the human face to the young child. He gets his first view of humanity from the face most closely associated with his first needs for food and contact.

The mother will try to elicit a response from the child, and if

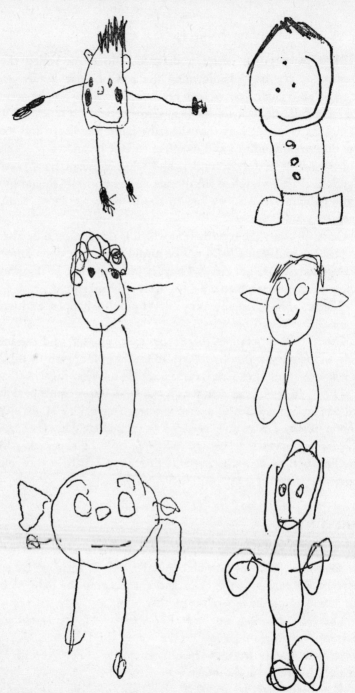

Examples of 4-year-old children's response to the Goodenough
'Draw a Man' Test.

the expected response does not come she may herself experience a feeling of rejection and begin to withdraw from the child.

If we can remember an occasion when we greeted a friend or acquaintance with a smile and it was not returned, we can see that even in adult life the significance of a response from the face of another is critical.

So all who have the care of a handicapped baby need to hold and support him so that he may look closely at the face of the person nearest, and begin to communicate with the world outside himself. He learns facial expressions by imitation and he interprets the world about him from the faces which surround him.

The infant receives active stimulation from the cuddling and caressing of his mother, and the mentally handicapped baby needs this more than most. Because he may be unusually passive, sleeping more than other babies, he may unwittingly be denied this essential care. The mother should be shown how to comfort and stimulate the baby at feeding and bathing times, how to support his head and move his limbs. If he has a 'floppy' side, that side needs extra careful stimulation. Many new mothers are afraid of hurting and handling the baby, fathers are more afraid of dropping the child and take a firm grip—babies prefer the feeling of security to tremulous clutching. Nurses need to spend time with the mother of a handicapped baby in a calm and unhurried way, so that the mother becomes involved early in what she can do to help the baby. The best time for this help is the very early days.

Care staff in maternity units, nursery nurses and other helpers, need to be shown how to help a mother with a handicapped baby right from the start, and this pattern of help should be firmly established before mother and baby return home.

Establishment of breast feeding may take longer if the baby is handicapped, especially if there is any abnormality of the nose or mouth. An extra large tongue, or blocked nasal airway will make it difficult for the baby to breathe as he sucks. Extra pillows help to support the mother in the best position, and to take the weight of the child so that she has both hands to free the nipple as far as possible, and to keep the baby's head back and the nasal passage clear as he feeds.

Because he is slower than others in some cases, he needs extra time for feeding, and routines designed for the majority of mothers may not suit him. His more prolonged and inefficient sucking may make the mother's nipples sore or she may have engorgement of insufficiently emptied breasts.

Comfort and care for the mother is essential, since her relationship with the infant must not be jeopardised in any way.

Most new babies cry a good deal—they need to exercise their newly acquired ability to breathe air. Mentally handicapped babies may cry much less than others, and so get less opportunity of lung expansion; or they may cry a great deal more, and fail to be comforted by usual means. Since continual crying is exhausting for the mother, the baby may be removed to a nursery so that she can sleep. If the baby is crying a good deal, he will be losing body fluids. Attention to temperature control is essential, and fluid replacement may be ordered.

Usually, the mother and baby will not return home from hospital until feeding is established and the birth weight regained. Staff of maternity units should ensure that the community nursing service and the general practitioner know when the mother and baby will return home, and that special help will be needed.

Once the early days are safely past and the baby is gaining weight satisfactorily—most babies seem to sleep better when they achieve a weight of around 10 lbs—the parents can begin to adjust to the demands of the new family member, and to initiate the special programme he will need.

Both can begin by discovering what he *can* do, and by asking for advice in designing a programme which will enable him to develop the inherent skills with which he was born, no matter how small these may be.

If the baby looks about him, even for very brief periods, the parents can present him with changes of light and shade, bright colours and glittering surfaces to engage his interest. If he can hear, he will enjoy tinkling sounds and musical notes.

Parents and helpers should not be tempted to continue stimulation by sight or sound over-long in order to elicit response. The primary need to build on success should always make early attempts stop short of failure. There is always another day. The handicapped baby is first and foremost a baby, and can be enjoyed as any baby is, for his own sake. Each day will bring new conditions, some good, some bad.

Mothers use a special 'language' when talking to a baby, repeating sounds and using a special intonation, often raising the pitch of their voice. Babies respond to this special tone, as if they understand from it that a particular communication is designed for them alone. Deprived of this special 'mothering language', babies become distressed or withdrawn and, if they are totally denied this verbal contact, will be unable to formulate speech sounds.

Mothers with very severely handicapped babies may not have the instinctive urge to make baby language sounds to them—feeling perhaps that if there is no response there is no value in the attempt to communicate. But the importance of the baby 'language' must be explained quietly, and the mother reassured that it is a truly positive contribution to his development.

HANDLING THE BABY

If the baby does not initiate the movements appropriate to his age—rolling, kicking, grasping, for instance—the mother will need to be shown how she can encourage these herself.

A firm surface at a comfortable height for her, covered with a thin layer of foam or other padding large enough to provide a good surface, will be most convenient for changing the baby and for exercise. A removable board which can be fixed over the bath, about 30 inches wide, can prove very useful if no other suitable surface is available. This is easily made secure by two solid battens on the underside, running parallel to the sides of the bath and set in slightly. The battens prevent the board from slipping into the bath when in use.

The bathroom should be warm whenever it is used for the baby; and every time he is changed or dressed, he should be exercised by extending the limbs, pulling him up by the arms, letting him feel the pushing of the mother's palm against the soles of his feet.

Later, the floor will be a more suitable surface for exercise play. The baby does need, and enjoy, regular warm bathing, and this too can give the chance of kicking and stretching exercises.

Some mentally handicapped babies have very dry and sensitive skins. It is best to avoid the use of quantities of talcum powder, and to use instead one of the pure baby oils to protect the skin. It may also be best to clean the buttocks with an oil-based baby lotion rather than with soap and water at every change.

Very sensitive skin may react to some synthetic fibres, and natural fibres of cotton or wool or a suitable mixture will give most comfort and adjust to skin temperature changes better than synthetics.

Care is also needed in the type of soap used, both for the baby's skin, and for washing his clothes. Biological-solvent type detergents should never be used to wash napkins or clothing and towels. However well they are washed and rinsed, they may retain enough of the active solvent to damage the skin. Pure soap flakes are probably best, and if any bleach is used, in soap powder or as a rinse for napkins, it must be very thoroughly rinsed out.

Such small details may seem trivial and obvious, but if the baby is a first baby, and particularly if the mother is not near family support and has no experience with babies, information on such basic care, shared with her by the nurse or helper, will give her a positive attitude to the care of the baby. These are things she can do whilst expert therapies are being arranged.

FEEDING

Breast feeding is naturally the best food for any baby, and every effort to help the mother to establish breast feeding successfully should be made. Natural antibodies in the milk protect the infant from many common infectious diseases, and this immunity will last through the first year if he is breast fed for the first months. By four or five months of age some weaning from breast or bottle can be commenced.

This should not be done too early. Either maternal milk or cow's milk (the latter with proper dilution and supplements) is perfectly adequate until the baby is between four and six months old. The first addition to the diet will be a cereal, probably a specially prepared baby cereal such as Farlene or Farex.

On the other hand many mentally handicapped babies and young children remain bottle fed far too long, with consequent damage to teeth. A single 'comfort' bottle once a day does no harm whatever, at any age, but the baby needs to be introduced early to semi-solid foods and the use of a spoon. The introduction of this first semi-solid food may be resisted, so it is most important that it should be gradual and pleasurable.

The quantity taken in this initial learning to feed from a spoon does not matter—the nutrition needs will still be being met by the milk feeds. But the methods used at this stage will condition future feeding success or failure. As feeding difficulties are high on the list of problems with handicapped children, we can spend a little time considering the best methods.

WEANING

First, the new food should be offered neither when the child is ravenously hungry, nor when he has had enough. Give part of the milk feed, and have ready a small quantity of mixed milk and cereal, warmed and standing in hot water to retain the temperature. In another small vessel have a plastic teaspoon—do not use a metal spoon, which may become too hot or too cold and has sharp edges.

On this spoon have ready a small blob of honey and offer this first, so that the baby associates the spoon with pleasure. When he sucks the honey efficiently, offer the smallest possible amount of the ceral food, gently closing his lips on it and softly encouraging swallowing by massaging the throat if he does not swallow.

If the baby is severely handicapped and swallowing is difficult, great patience will be needed, and the infant may do no more to start with than accept the honey. Even this is a start. Do not give up if the spoon is totally rejected, but leave it for another day, and continue with the bottle feed. Perseverance with feeding from a spoon and later a cup, from the earliest months, is another positive step forward and will repay all the patient effort.

SLEEPING

Many handicapped babies have disturbed sleep patterns, crying or rocking at night and disturbing the sleep of both parents. The mother thus needs to be encouraged to take her rest during the day whenever the child sleeps, and not to use these periods to catch up on household tasks. One benefit of breast feeding is that the mother must rest as she feeds the child. She can be advised to lie down with the child to do so, and to sleep afterwards.

If the father has to work all day the burden of disturbed sleep will place a further strain on the family, and it may sometimes be best to make a temporary arrangement for him to sleep elsewhere in the house, even the living room, until a sleep pattern is achieved.

Disturbed sleep can become a problem for some years of childhood so the help of the family doctor should be sought at an early stage if the baby shows no sign of settling to an acceptable pattern.

Mothers may frequently be fearful of leaving a young baby to the care of anyone else, and sometimes the mother of a handicapped baby rejects any help because she feels an overwhelming sense of responsibility for the child. If help is refused when it is most needed, for whatever reason, it may set a pattern of isolation for mother and child which will be very difficult to break. Parents should thus be encouraged to take help whenever it is offered, once a daily routine has been established which can be carried out by another person. Even one night or day free of the demands of the child may be enough to restore the energies of the parents.

FRESH AIR

The out of doors—even in a city—provides a change of scene, for the mother no less than the baby, and helpers need to support and encourage the mother not only to make use of the garden, if there is one, but to start early to take the baby outside the home for walks. However, many modern baby chairs and prams are arranged so that the child has his back to the mother and she cannot see his face as they walk. They are also too near the ground, the baby sees nothing but feet, pavements and the wheels of traffic. If there is any choice, babies are much happier in the old high pram, facing the mother, so that she can talk to him and increase his awareness of sunshine, trees, rain, and other features of his environment.

IMPROVING MUSCLE TONE

If the baby is carried in a sling, avoid those which have a wide strap between the legs and force the hips apart and the legs to dangle. The mentally handicapped baby has poor muscle tone and needs support. Similarly, when he is put down into a cot or pram to sleep, avoid putting him on his stomach. This position is often used in hospital nurseries with the baby prone and the face turned to one side because there is less risk of an unsupervised baby choking if he regurgitates food. There are considerable disadvantages in that if this position is maintained too long, the ankles are dropped and kicking is inhibited. The use of stretch one-piece suits also restricts movements of the toes if they are not really large and loose. The result of a combination of too-long lying on the belly and too small one-piece stretch suits is the tip-toe posture seen in some small children as they start to walk.

Babies with good muscle tone may soon correct this, but mentally handicapped babies need every help possible to *prevent* poor habits adding to their disabilities. Warm, loose clothing, every opportunity for independent movement, the encouragement of all natural kicking, rolling and head movements are essential.

SITTING

So that he can make the most of the learning potential of his surroundings, the baby needs to be supported in a sitting position as often as possible. If the parents carry him in their arms, for instance, in a sitting position, the firm support and closeness of contact will give him confidence to look about him.

Every time he turns his head to see new objects, to follow the movement of leaves on trees or reflections of light on water, he is strengthening the muscles which support his head and preparing them for more movements. He can be propped with cushions in the corner of an armchair to watch his mother in her daily tasks, or on the floor by means of foam pieces. At all times try to keep the mid-line of the body straight and the limbs well supported. Prolonged use of some types of moulded shell supports, however, if they are not individually designed, can contract the limbs into poor patterns, and some walking aids which suspend the baby in a sling seat, swinging with feet barely touching the ground, are dangerous, too. Periods of relaxing and swinging, being tossed up in the air, if he enjoys this, or being held under the arms to test the sensation of taking weight on his feet, can be stimulating, but all such activities need to be varied and purposeful.

At this very early stage, the mother needs all the guidance and support possible. Nurses and care staff should never assume that mothering is natural and that she will know by instinct what to do. Mothering practices are imitative, and are learned, so if a mother has already had other children she will indeed use the experience and skill learned on the earlier child. If she has younger brothers and sisters, she will have watched her own mother care for them and will probably have helped with their care. But the mother without these experiences needs help with even the simplest practices. We hear well known personalities on the television screen admit that returning home with a baby to care for terrified them in a way that the most demanding public appearance did not.

If the baby is handicapped, these feelings of inadequacy and real terror at being left to cope can overwhelm the mother.

Quiet practical advice on everyday care, which results in a good daily rhythm and some reasonable degree of rest within the first few weeks, can be a life-line, and nurses and helpers need to feel confident themselves, so that they can support the mother, without taking over her caring role. Confidence comes with successful achievement, so nurses and helpers can design the steps which are most productive of good results, and can then wait for the mother to decide what she and the baby should tackle next.

Much time has been spent in discussing the very early weeks of life because in this period the brain is developing fast and patterns are imprinted which can be beneficial or harmful for years to come. Prevention of patterns and habits which will block future progress is thus more important than achievement at this stage.

THE TWO-YEAR-OLD AND TODDLER

We can pass, in this small handbook, rapidly from the health aspects of caring for the very young baby to the two-year-old because we can get excellent help from Health Visitors at this early period and advice from clinic staff. Detailed studies of the way babies grow and develop have been described in a number of excellent books, listed in the Bibliography, so we shall only introduce the topic and set out the general principles.

By two years most handicapped babies will make attempts to sit alone, make a recognisable sound for 'mother', be able to fit simple toys together, respond to sounds, and show pleasure or displeasure in a recognisable way. How much else he can do will depend upon his abilities and even more upon what opportunity he has had to learn.

He will weigh approximately four times his birthweight—around 12·5 kgms.—and be ready to accept short separations from his mother and to play in a group with other children.

Play group

Most areas where there are several mothers with young children will now have a play group within reach, and mentally handicapped children can join with children without handicaps with advantage to each.

Play group leaders may be mothers themselves and some may have taken special training in the running of the groups. Toys of many different types are provided.* Some are designed for gross motor play to strengthen large muscles and improve balance and posture, others such as small puzzles and toys which need to be fitted together, encourage hand-eye co-ordination. There may also be water play, painting, dressing up, soft toys to cuddle. Each session will be planned to give some time to each activity.

Milk or fruit juice, biscuits or fruit may be offered in the course of the session, and in some cases all the children may share a main meal.

To begin with, the child should not be left at the group session. The mother or helper should remain with him, letting him stay close until he feels secure enough to join other small children.

The child is continuing his social learning, outside his home, and will experience frustration and satisfaction in his interaction with others. He will also, by imitation of the actions of other children more able than he, find models of new skills.

Common infections

There will be a greater risk of common infections when the child joins a group, and the mother will need to be alert to the signs of common illnesses and to take appropriate care.

The various protective immunisations available at the local child clinics will be offered at three months on, and the two-year-old will be protected against some of the common ailments.

Recommended Ages for Protective Immunisation

3 months	Diphtheria 1	Separately or Combined
	Tetanus 1	
	Whooping Cough 1	
	Polio 1	
5 months	Diphtheria 2	Separately or Combined
	Tetanus 2	
	Whooping Cough 2	
	Polio 2	

*Many on loan from Toy Libraries, which also lend to other institutions and to individual families. (See Resource List.)

9 months	Diphtheria 3 Tetanus 3 Whooping Cough 3 Polio 3	Separately or Combined
12 months	Measles	
When starting school	Diphtheria 4 Tetanus 4 Polio 4	Combined
13 years	TB (Tuberculosis)	If not immune
11–13 years	German Measles (Rubella)	Girls only
When leaving school	Tetanus 5 Polio 5	

Coughs and colds are very common in the winter months, and the handicapped baby cannot entirely escape them. It is wise to avoid very crowded places where a mixture of infections is likely, especially if the child is already off colour.

Small children run high temperatures very quickly as a response to infection, become irritable or lethargic, lose appetite, have bowel or sleep disturbances.

Sometimes they recover with equal rapidity—the temperature falling to normal within a very short time—which can be embarrassing if the doctor has been summoned to a house call. So a useful rule is that *one* abnormal symptom may not be very serious, but if two or more are present help should be sought. If there is evidence of a raised temperature *and* the child shows signs of pain, ear-ache or colic, for example, treatment is urgently indicated.

If in doubt, seek the doctor's advice. It is better to be wrong than to leave a condition until it is critical.

If it is known that he has been in contact with an infectious disease, the mother may care to know how long it may be before signs of symptoms arise.

Usual periods are:

Infectious Diseases

Short Incubation Periods

	Incubation Period	Infectious for	Quarantine Period
Scarlet Fever and other Streptococcal Infections	1–3 days	A few days before onset until free of symptoms	On advice of doctor
Meningoccal Infections	2–10 days average 3–4	Whilst organism present in nose and throat	On advice of doctor
Diphtheria	2–5 days	Whilst organism is present in nose and throat	On advice of doctor
Poliomyelitis	3–21 days average 7–12	From 36 hours before onset and whilst virus present in stools	On advice of doctor

Long Incubation Periods

Chicken Pox	14–21 days average 13–17	1 day before to 6 days after rash	7 days after rash disappears
Measles	10 days to onset of illness then 10 days to onset of rash	4 days before to 5 days after rash appears	On advice of doctor

	Incubation Period	Infectious for	Quarantine Period
German Measles (Rubella)	14–21 days	4–5 days after catarrhal symptoms	4–5 days after rash disappears

Long Incubation Periods

	Incubation Period	Infectious for	Quarantine Period
Mumps	12–26 days average 18	7 days before to 9 days after swelling appears	On advice of doctor
Whooping Cough	7–10 days Not more than 21	From early stage to 3 weeks after 'whoop' commenced	Until 3 weeks after whooping starts

Infectious diseases pass through the stages of incubation, when the disease is not noticeable but may infect others; the open or active state when the specific signs of the disease show themselves, for example a rash or cough; and a stage of healing. At all these stages others may be infected. The severity of an attack will be affected by the health of the person, the severity of the infection, and the care received whilst he is ill.

In general, all fevers of childhood require good home-nursing care, so that a second complication may not supervene on the original disease: pneumonia upon whooping cough, ear infections after measles and so on.

Nursing care is designed to assist the body's own healing by providing rest, suitable diet—usually plenty of fluids—avoidance of chills or over-heating and adequate rest and sleep. The sick child will often decide for himself whether he wishes to remain in bed or be quietly occupied in the living room. He will certainly need extra comforting and the relief of symptoms peculiar to the disease.

Symptoms of common fevers

Measles. Often preceded by a period of running nose, sore eyes and general misery before the rash is seen. The common complications are discharging ears, dislike of light—the child may demand a darkened room.

German Measles. Often only a slightly stiff neck, some enlargement of the glands of the neck and back of the head, and a bright small rash appearing very quickly and fading equally fast. It is a very mild disease *BUT* it is exceedingly dangerous to pregnant women in the first stages of pregnancy because it may result in a damaged baby. Be very careful to keep a child with German measles (*Rubella*) away from pregnant women.

Mumps. Painful swelling of the parotid gland—the gland at the angle of the jaw. The child may cry if he tastes an acid fruit drink, as this causes a spasm of the salivary gland. Once the swelling begins, the diagnosis is obvious. The infection may spread to other glands, ovaries or testicles, and again, it is wise to keep the child away from adults who may not have had the disease.

Chicken Pox. A rash of small blisters which forms in the creases of the abdomen, neck, wrists or knees, and on the face. It is intensely irritating and the child may pick and scratch himself severely.

Baths to which soda bicarbonate have been added will help to induce sleep at bedtime, and a paste of soda bicarbonate will relieve itching during the day. The child should be distracted from scratching, as the spots may become infected and cause scarring as they heal. Chicken pox can be passed to adults and may then cause shingles, which in older people can be very painful and take months to cure.

Two diseases which must not be considered trivial are whooping cough and diphtheria.

Whooping cough results in acute spasms of coughing in which the child cannot breathe properly. He may become blue in the face and the heart is subjected to great strain in the coughing bouts. He will usually vomit after a bout of coughing, and so become very exhausted and dehydrated. If the child becomes ill with whooping cough the doctor's advice should be sought at once.

Protection is available in the form of a vaccine. This vaccine has been suspected, in some cases, of causing damage. The number of cases of proven connection is small, but significant enough for each parent to consider carefully the arguments for and against protection.

Diphtheria. This disease has been almost completely eradicated by protective immunisation. Before the protection was available, babies died every year from the membrane which formed at the back of the throat and choked the child. It is a rare disease now, but if any suspicion of contact with a case occurs, perhaps after travel abroad, advice must be sought.

Mothers and helpers will certainly come in contact with one or more of these diseases during the childhood of the baby. In the case of most of them, one attack will bring life-long immunity from repetition, and early recognition of the symptoms and prompt treatment will usually ensure that they pass without much harm.

SECTION NINE

The School Years

The School Years

The handicapped baby may be admitted to some form of education—in a nursery class, or with an individual teacher—as early as two years if he is in an area with good provisions. Particularly if he has already been in a play group, he will be ready to learn and to profit by wider experience.

The nursery school years will bring him into contact with other children and with the trained teachers who can devise a special learning environment for his individual needs. The nurses and helpers who have been so central to his world up to this point, ensuring that his physical and emotional needs are met, can now stand aside a little. It is very important however to provide continuity and to see that everyone works together for the benefit of the child, so the school group, wherever it is situated, will need help from the parents or care staff to ensure that their work is most effective.

The child needs to arrive at school fresh, not over-tired by insufficient sleep; properly clothed so that he is neither chilled or too warm; and properly fed.

At all schools for handicapped children, nursing and medical supervision is provided by the School Health Service, and some nurses find this work very rewarding.

All the responsibilities we have already described for staff in other institutions also apply to the school nurse. She looks for early identification of medical problems, such as defects of sight or hearing; she observes the children as they arrive for signs of illness; she notes the general environment of the school from the point of view of health; and she deals with emergencies and gives first aid if needed. She will also note the progress of any children under special medical treatment. Her task is to support the educational work by a partnership of skill, and she is often a valuable means of liaison among the home, the school, the family doctor, and other specialists. The child is still in a rapidly formative period and early intervention to deal with adverse conditions as soon as they are noted is vital.

Social workers giving family support may also be involved in cases where the child is needing special care; and they will always be involved if the child is not living with his family. They will attend the medical examinations and give information to the doctor or nurse, and give back information to the residential care staff. In some areas there is a rapid staff turnover among social workers, which may complicate the treatment of a child with a continuing physical disability, and in such cases the school nurse may be able to act as an extra support by, for instance, making a personal liaison with the residential home.

Though the child spends many hours each day away from home, there are still periods of school holidays, weekends and the hours at home to consider, so residential staff and helpers as well as parents continue to be crucial to his progress.

When the child begins his full school day he will undoubtedly be tired, and this may exaggerate behaviour problems which appear to have been solved much earlier. He may become incontinent again, and need patient reassurance and a return to the original training programmes. His sleep may be disturbed, and he may wake with fears and dreams and need to be quickly comforted and reassured.

If he has had a change of environment connected with school attendance—for example, be living in a residential school during the week—there may be considerable disturbance, and liaison between his home, school and residential staff is essential.

DISTURBED BEHAVIOUR

The result of emotional upset may be very disturbed behaviour. It is important to understand that, if a child cannot put his fears into words or otherwise communicate them to adults around him, he will react by attention-seeking behaviour.

This may begin as an exaggeration of comforting practices, such as rocking himself. He will have enjoyed the rhythm of being rocked and soothed as a baby, and may revert to it as a means of comfort in alarming situations. If he does not receive the attention and comfort he needs, the rocking may become more and more prolonged, and be continued into head-banging or other self-damaging practices.

He may develop ritual behaviour, or return to a pattern of this type which has previously been passed. Holding a particular toy or object and reacting violently if it is removed is one example of this type of self-comforting behaviour. In a final, extreme form the child may withdraw completely and sit alone in a corner, or even curl up into the foetal position and refuse to move. All these types of behaviour are his defences against a threatening world and are as clear an indication that he needs help as if he communicated it in words.

More violent reactions may result in damaging toys or home equipment, screaming and over-active behaviour, running or jumping about without purpose. Such behaviour is very disturbing to a group of children or to a family, and needs much patience to deal with it.

If it is understood that the child is asking for help to deal with a situation which he cannot manage himself, not just being naughty or deliberately troublesome, it will be seen that reassurance is the first step. This can be given by letting the child see that he is still approved of—though his behaviour is not. If the destructive behaviour, rocking or screaming, is rewarded with instant attention, it will continue, so the helper or parents is in a serious dilemma : if the behaviour is ignored it becomes worse, and if rewarded, it will be constantly repeated. An expert may well have to be brought in to help break the vicious circle.

Some general principles may however be helpful. First discover what triggers off the behaviour, trace the situation which causes fear, identify factors which provoke boredom or anger, and then eliminate or reduce these. If the child is afraid of steps or stairs for example, he can be encouraged to play upon firm brightly coloured boxes in the play group or physical education class, with much help, until he overcomes his fear of falling. Fears of this kind spring from his inability to appreciate spatial relationships—when a surface is flat or when vertical, and how to adapt his movements to deal with the changing levels.

Fears of the dark, of awakening in a strange place, may trigger off apparently unrelated behaviour which is very hard to understand. But time spent quietly analysing what causes the disturbance will help to devise methods of preventing or reducing it.

Once a pattern of disturbed behaviour is set it is more difficult to eradicate, so the next principle is to watch carefully for signs that it is about to occur, and immediately offer a distraction.

Severe bouts of rocking and head banging must be checked immediately. This may involve sitting with the child and physically preventing the action by immobilising him, whilst talking to him in a quiet reassuring fashion. When he is released and does not resume the disturbed behaviour, he should be immediately rewarded with a smile, a hug, a very small sweet or other specially enjoyed treat; and immediately given some personal activity which he enjoys.

Treating this type of behaviour is immensely time-consuming and exhausting for the helper, and it may be necessary for one person to have no other duty until the behaviour has been eradicated or reduced to manageable levels. Sometimes the eradication of one type of disturbed behaviour results in the child developing another self-comforting pattern which has to be patiently dealt with again.

Severely disturbed behaviour prevents any learning and so must be dealt with before any other help can be given. Special behaviour modification programmes may be needed, and expert help should be sought.

All such behaviour is symptomatic of inner distress and cries out for help. Identification of the cause may be difficult, since it may have no obvious connection with outside stimulus at all, perhaps the result of confusion in perception. Whether the cause is understood or not, treatment is designed to bring comfort and relief, and each child will need help suited to his particular temperament and to the patterns he had received in his earlier care.

SAFETY

The handicapped child may have no personal sense of danger, and parents and helpers have to anticipate perils for him at ages long past those when fearlessness of physical harm is a normal feature of childhood.

Very young children will often climb quite dangerous structures in their desire to learn and experience what they can achieve. They have no fear of fire until they are burned, and do not understand that electrical appliances can give shocks. But experience will teach them to avoid what can hurt them.

The severely retarded child, however, is not capable of the same degree of transferred learning as normal children.

Parents with mentally handicapped children at home have usually developed safety routines which protect the child well in his home environment. They also may have taught him to cross a road beside his home perfectly safely, because the familiar practice has become a routine, learned by continuous exercise. But he may be totally confused by the need to cross a strange road, where landmarks such as letter boxes and traffic islands are in a different place.

Similarly, he may be unable to perform tasks in a new environment which he can perform perfectly well at home. Lavatories, handbasins in unfamiliar surroundings are, to him, totally new territory. He needs much more time to transfer what he can do in one situation to a new one, because for him, this involves new learning.

When we are faced with a new situation we deal with it not only by marshalling past experience, but by a logical selection of information, discarding and retaining until we are using only the elements of learned behaviour needed for the new circumstances. We often do this so fast that we are not even aware of the process. Most of us continue to use a handbasin anywhere, no matter how different the plumbing arrangements—though some of those encountered when travelling abroad may take some working out!

If we can analyse this type of situation when we experience it personally, it may help us to understand the confusion and dis-

tress experienced by a mentally handicapped child confronted
with too many new experiences at one time.

Helpers and care staff need to understand this and to be alert to
make changes as simple as possible, and to check at all times that
unfamiliar routines are free from danger.

ENCOURAGEMENT

Since the whole object of education is to develop the potential
gifts of the child and to lead him towards independence, we
protect and comfort him only so far as is needed to make him
receptive to learning.

He cannot learn if he is distressed or confused, so that must
be dealt with first. But that done, every opportunity of contact
with the child can be used either to increase his confidence or
further to erode it. It is important to be aware of the difference.

Small skills learned, putting on socks and shoes, for example,
if they are promptly rewarded, build confidence and lead to progress. The 'comfort' of having someone always doing things for
the child, however, may have the opposite effect.

In the residential situation, individual assessment of capabilities
and designed opportunities to use and develop them are as essential as in school.

Equally, the child is learning to be part of a group, to subju-
gate some of what he wants to do to the wants of others. Care staff
have thus the added responsibility to make the advantages of
conformity plain to handicapped children, and as these are by no
means always plain even to the non-handicapped this again needs
a lively imagination and original approach.

On the other hand if the structured activities at school are
carefully controlled to provide the best learning conditions, home
is often the place for letting off steam, for relaxation. Since this
need is as great for the handicapped child as for others, a good
routine will allow for periods which supply this need. But staff
need to be sensitive to the need to intervene occasionally.

The child will enjoy free play, but because his imagination is
limited his activity may become stereotyped and meaningless if he

is not helped. He may turn the pages of a book for long periods without understanding. Such activities may be part of his 'unwinding', pleasurable in themselves and should not be interfered with unless they show signs of becoming a fixed ritual which interferes with activities which have more opportunities for learning.

Most children at school quickly discover that some activities are better shared—games and dressing up for instance—and this knowledge helps them to adapt to sharing activities at home. Some children however need help in learning to share.

Care staff need above all to observe the child as an individual in order to supply his needs in the school years.

ACCIDENTS

Prevention

Most accidents occur in the home, and many are preventable. The adage that 'accidents don't happen, they are caused' is still true.

Burns and scalds are a hazard of the kitchen, so very young children and children so retarded as to be unable to protect themselves should not be in the kitchen when cooking is going on and the attention of mother or helper is elsewhere.

A small gate across the door may allow the child to see the mother as he plays, and keep him from harm. Electric kettles must be used only on surfaces well away from small hands, hot drinks and teapots are best used without a table cloth which can be pulled by a child.

All helpers and staff should put cold water *first* into a bath intended for a child, adding hot water until the desired temperature is reached. They should then test the water before introducing the child. If this practice is adopted as routine, the danger of scalding because the child gets into too hot a bath before he is told to do so, or helped into it, is minimised.

Care is needed whenever hot water is used for cleaning and laundry work, and care staff will arrange routines to minimise the dangers of burns and scalds.

Fire hazards involve asphyxiation by fumes as well as burns,

especially when man-made synthetics are involved, such as poly-
ester fibres used in upholstery, fabrics and mattresses.

Special care should be taken that even when fire guards are in
place nothing can fall or be placed over a source of heat.

Sharp knives, tins, glass, are all possible hazards, and in the
family situation frequent cause of accidents. Articles such as toys,
dustpans and other cleaning equipment left on stairs cause falls
and fractures.

Electric socket outlets need to be of the safety guarded type,
which will not allow the child to poke small implements into
them. Trailing electric flex too is a danger.

First aid

There are a few life-threatening accidents which require immediate aid.

Asphyxia, whether from choking or drowning, is one of these.
If a child is found to have stopped breathing for any reason,
urgent action is indicated. The air-way must be cleared, the
tongue brought forward and artificial respiration commenced. A
small child may be held upside down by the heels first and given
a sharp blow between the shoulders, before being placed in the
position for the kiss of life.

To give the kiss of life, hold the nose pinched to close the
nostrils, then place your mouth over that of the child, breathe
gently into the child's mouth to inflate the lungs, and release the
pressure on the nose to allow exhalation. If there is any means of
summoning the aid of a second person by shouting or calling, do so,
so that transport to hospital can be swiftly organised. All measures
to restore breathing must continue until professional help arrives.
This technique must be learnt *practically*, and a member of staff
should be fully conversant with life-saving techniques.

Severe bleeding from an injury is also life-threatening, and
urgent help may be needed. If a limb is involved, raise it above the
level of the heart: if it is a hand or arm lift it above the head
whilst maintaining pressure on the bleeding part; if a leg, lay the
person down and raise the leg, applying pressure on and above
the bleeding point.

Head wounds frequently bleed very profusely; and all head injuries and severe injuries result in shock. If the person faints or becomes unconscious he will fall naturally, if he does not, he must be kept lying down until professional help is obtained. Do not allow a child who has received a head injury to walk about until professional help arrives. First aid for any but the most trivial accidents is best given at a hospital, and time should not be wasted by any amateur help except in life-threatening situations.

Minor accidents however can be dealt with at home by first cleaning the wound gently with soap and water, drying as far as possible with clean linen or cotton wool, applying a simple dressing—vaseline, Friar's Balsam, or a proprietary antiseptic cream—and covering with a suitable adhesive dressing or bandage. Bumps and bruises are quickly relieved with a compress—a soaked pad of linen—of witch hazel lotion.

More elaborate dressings and drugs are not needed. The home first aid box need contain only a few essentials, but these *must* always be replaced. Suggested basic essentials are: a large jar of vaseline; a bottle of witch hazel; a bottle of Friar's Balsam; a box of elastic adhesive dressings; a few cotton bandages; clean washed old linen in squares or strips, or white lint; cotton wool; a pair of scissors; a simple antiseptic cream.

Small burns are best placed immediately under a running cold tap until the pain is relieved. Repeat the process if the smarting commences again. Scalds on arms or legs can be given this first aid cold water treatment in a bath. But all severe scalds and burns need hospital care.

Poisons

Common dangers in a home are cleaning fluids, laundry requisites, disinfectants and medicines prescribed for others.

In the lavatory and bathroom, make sure that all cleaning agents are kept off the floor—high above the reach of children. Kitchen cleaning items also need to be well out of their reach.

Garden chemicals can be lethal, do not have them in the house at all and keep them locked outside.

All medicines are a danger to young children and none should be stored where they can be reached.

If any harmful product is taken by a child, it is most important to take the bottle or other container with the child to hospital and to give some idea of the quantity taken. Do not waste time looking for antidotes, get the child to a hospital.

It is mainly in childhood and early adult life that accidents occur, and their possibility must be anticipated and as far as possible prevented by those responsible for care. Remember always when caring for mentally handicapped children that they have great difficulty in transferring learning from one situation to another—they will not be able to anticipate danger from a different hazard, even if they have experienced hurt from a similar source.

Fortunately, in some respects they are protected to a degree by their relatively low level of curiosity, but helpers must anticipate real dangers, whilst encouraging adventure into new situations and allowing the child to learn by mistakes.

SECTION TEN

Puberty and Adolescence

Social Education

Continued Education

Sexual Behaviour

Life Skills

Special Disabilities

Leisure

Puberty and Adolescence

In many ways, the school years of the child are a period of reasonable stability. There may have been episodes of illness or accident, of emotional upset due to change in the environment, changes in family life or of staff which affect the child, but in general the middle years of childhood are contained within the provisions of the educational service, which, in comparison with other community services, is well organised and well provided. Assessment for special education, monitoring of physical disabilities and flexibility in the type of school or teacher advised for the child is available everywhere in greater or lesser degrees.

At around the age of twelve years—sometimes younger for girls and later for boys—puberty commences. Severely retarded children may have the normal ages of onset of physical maturity delayed, but the signs of developing sexuality are usually noted early in the second decade of life.

There is a growth spurt, which makes demands on the body in a physical sense : more sleep is often needed, the lengthening of the long bones may increase poor co-ordination difficulties so that the child becomes more clumsy and awkward. Diet needs attention to provide the proteins needed for growth, and dental care is important at this stage, as the permanent teeth are now being completed and aligned as the jaw develops to the adult size.

But far more important to the helpers and family are the emotional changes which mark this period of life. Triggered by the hormonal output of the glands, an upheaval of the comparative calm of childhood commences, and the personality enters a period of storm and stress.

Every child, handicapped or not, is subject to this process, and the effects are in direct relation to his environment and to patterns set during his childhood.

In ordinary circumstances, the child adjusts daily to the changes within himself, which he cannot fully understand, by behaviour designed to relieve his inner tensions. His personal methods may vary.

Some children will insist on a privacy which they have not so far demanded, they may lock themselves in a room of their own, or demand a room to themselves when they have previously happily shared with another child. To withdraw from the group, especially a group composed of people of mixed ages, as in a family, seems to become an essential need for some young people in order to come to terms with their own developing personalities.

Others seem to deliberately provoke confrontation situations with adults, by defying and challenging rules and customs which they had previously accepted without trouble.

Mentally handicapped young people will experience all the turbulence and distress of the adolescent period in greater or lesser degree and express it by changes in behaviour just like other youngsters!

Sexuality develops in everyone; how much it is a driving force in personality differs from one person to another, male or female, and the same is true of mentally handicapped people.

Curiosity about the physical signs of development are natural : pubic hair, voice changes, breast and genital enlargement; and exploring these changes is a method of learning.

There is also now a whole new code of appropriate behaviour to be learned, and mentally handicapped young adults may well be bewildered by social customs which cause trouble enough to young people without this handicap. They are no longer children, but they are not yet adults, and will not be adults, physically, for several years.

Hormonal changes will continue, and the delicate balance needed for effective body function will take years to achieve. The hormones control emotional moods, as well as physical growth, and if the mentally handicapped child has been maintained in childhood on drugs to stabilise emotional reactions, the changed hormonal output will also disorganise this routine.

Behaviour problems which had been contained by careful conditioning in early childhood may now commence again; and frustrations arising from the impossibility of understanding what is happening may erupt into violent behaviour, usually directed at parents or other adults in a hitherto unchallenged position of authority.

What can be done to help young people through this stage? Before we can decide, we need some knowledge of what is common to everyone at this time in their lives, and some understanding of the effects on the mentally handicapped.

Many adults cannot remember their own feelings at this time in their lives, because it was so traumatic that a merciful sponge has wiped it from adult memory; but some of us can still recall something of the experience.

One characteristic of adolescence is a heightened awareness of the world around, as though suddenly one sees with new eyes. This results in both heightened pleasure and greater pain, so helpers in contact with mentally handicapped young people— parents, teachers, social workers—must expect extremes of behaviour and sharpened sensitivities, and try to deal with each as they come.

The awakening of sexuality however also results in a more alert interest in the world in general, as well as in the particular, because human sexuality is part of the whole personality, not confined to reproduction alone.

This in effect provides a 'second chance' to educate, to awaken curiosity, develop individual potential and form a pattern of adult behaviour which can be a basis for life.

Mentally handicapped people may well have a much longer period of adolescence than others, so would benefit from a longer period of structured education. Compulsory education ceases at 16 years in the United Kingdom, but mentally handicapped young people may receive continued secondary education beyond this period, based upon their needs, and upon parental demand for it.

The continuation of skills and acquisition of new social skills is so important to mentally handicapped people that everyone caring for them should be aware of what is available, and try to ensure that what is needed is provided.

SOCIAL EDUCATION

By virtue of their handicap and their need of support in child-hood, many mentally handicapped children have led compara-tively sheltered lives. In residential schools or in the home, they have often been cut off from the world of shopping, using public transport, telephone and similar community amenities. Nor has training for careers and subsequent employment usually been part of the planned curriculum either in the final school years for them, or in any special Further Education service.

Instead, the mentally handicapped school leaver leaves a com-paratively calm and organised system just at the time when he most needs support.

Change and challenge is an essential learning condition for normal young people. They are equipped to deal with it by their varying ability to select from past experience and to predict the probable results of new experience. They are adjusting daily, comparing fresh information with old, accumulating and evalua-ting, with whatever difficulty, the changing circumstances of their lives.

For this process, the mentally handicapped young adult is ill-equipped. He is slow, change bewilders him, he has to repeat new techniques and new experiences dozens of times before they are absorbed, and he has no store of basic scientific learning, for example, to help him to understand his own personality changes, nor can he reason logically or predict from past experience.

Parents and staff can help in a number of practical ways. They can ensure that any medication is reviewed regularly, and they can ensure that adequate rest is obtained—even if this means that the adolescent sleeps on longer in the morning, or sleeps in the day because he wishes to stay up later at night. They can accept that the company of other young people of his own age is more important and more helpful to him than theirs, and they can allow him an increasing degree of independence to make mis-takes, then help him to analyse and learn from them.

Each young person is an individual. Some will have so calm a personality that they pass almost unnoticed from adolescence into adult life; some will have so stormy a passage that they may become temporarily in need of specialist medical or psychiatric care. But in accordance with their ability all need social education to acquire if possible sufficient skills to manage their own daily life. They need to manage their own clothing—purchasing clothes suitable for the weather, for instance; to make simple meals and purchase the requirements; to understand local transport; and to know where to go for help in emergencies, at the very least. Some will be able to read sufficiently to understand commonly encountered public instructions, some will be numerate and understand money, some will have special skills of value to the community.

Others will need maximum supervision all their lives, for their own safety and that of others, and these young people will probably be cared for in small residential group homes with specially trained staff.

CONTINUED EDUCATION

There is increasing acceptance of the need for both general and occupational education for mentally handicapped adults, and in some areas courses both full- and part-time are available through the Further Education system.

Some special training establishments give social education and vocational training on a residential basis and accept mentally handicapped young people leaving school for periods of up to two years. They are taught skills for future employment, life skills or self-care and how to manage their relationships with others.

Education of this kind is also provided in hospital units for severely retarded people with additional handicaps, and some social services departments organise practical training for residents in group homes and sheltered housing.

Young adults are keen for new experience, but the restlessness typical of this age group may make them unwilling to concentrate for long periods on subjects which do not immediately interest them. So professional teaching skills and experience should look for methods of holding attention, of giving only as much information as can be absorbed at one time, and of providing opportunities to use new skills.

Care staff, and nursing staff of hospitals, need to work closely with the teaching staff and to become teachers themselves in their role of caring for the young adult. In any case, a trained teacher is not always available.

Any teaching session, be it academic—passing on such skills as literarcy or numeracy—or practical—showing a young man how to use a razor, for example—must be structured for best results. It is most helpful if there is a good friendly relationship already established between the two partners in learning, and if the skill to be learned is a desired skill on the part of the student, though this is not always possible.

The first requirement for effective learning is that the programme be designed within the capacity of understanding of the student. If we illustrate this with the example of shaving, a mentally handicapped young man needs to have sufficient co-ordination to use an electric razor, but he does not need to understand in the least the principles of electric voltages. He can be instructed *at his level*, and the helper has the responsibility of ensuring that he is sufficiently aware of any inherent dangers.

The next requirement is to achieve the full attention of the student. Many mentally handicapped people are very distractable, and to gain their attention may mean removing them from a group and into surroundings which do not offer distraction. Small rooms may be available for individual instruction in schools and other buildings, but if no purpose-built room is available, the existing environment and routine must be adjusted to provide this one-to-one situation.

The identification of exactly what has to be taught is the next step, and a decision made about precisely how much can be learned at one time. The use of the electric razor, to go back to our example, may be familiar to the young man because he has seen others using one; but if it is totally a new experience, the teacher will need to think himself into the position of the student, then work out how the process can be broken down into suitable steps, and how much practice will be required to perfect the skill.

Hair styling for young women, using make-up or other cosmetics, care of the feet and choice of shoes will all need to be approached in a similar way.

Patience and interest will be required of whoever is in the teaching role. Parents and care staff who have known the young person through his childhood will obviously be most familiar with what methods are likely to prove successful with a particular youngster: but just as ordinary children tend to leave the childhood home in early adult life, so, increasingly, mentally handicapped young people will change their established life-style at this age, and some care staff and helpers will be confronted with young people already confused by a move from their previous home. A period of adjustment to this change is very necessary, and some disturbed behaviour should be allowed for.

Many Education Authorities now offer courses both full- and part-time designed for mentally handicapped young adults. Others are currently planning for these provisions. Some register mentally handicapped students with others in Further Education courses or Adult Education courses from which they can profit. A list of courses currently available appears in Anne Henshaw's *After Sixteen*, listed in the Bibliography. Parents and staff members should enquire at their Local Education office about the availability of courses in their own area, and study the prospectus of local colleges of further education to see if there are appropriate courses for which their young adults could be enrolled alongside ordinary young people.

Some examples of courses shared by mentally handicapped people and others are cookery classes, reading and numeracy classes, floral arrangement, woodwork, social skills and work introduction courses.

SEXUAL BEHAVIOUR

Probably nothing causes more difficulty at this stage of life than awakening sexuality and its expression. The severely mentally handicapped young adult will experience the sensations associated with sexual maturity and the biological manifestations, no less than others, but the reactions of both young men and young women will differ from those of their more able peers.

Ordinary young people have been conditioned from childhood to understand community attitudes to sexuality—whether they conform to them or not. If they deviate from accepted social behaviour they do so consciously, and are aware of the possible consequences. They also understand the implications of their social behaviour—for example, that promiscuity has dangers to the individual and consequences to the community—so they can make informed choices about what they do.

Mentally handicapped young adults cannot function at this reasoning level. They have probably always been familiar with the pleasurable sensations evoked by stroking or fondling, and have sought them or rejected them according to their temperament. But now the urgency to gratify sexual urges is increased, and those who in childhood indulged only in occasional masturbation may do so with increased frequency and intensity. It provides a release from physical tension for both men and women and does no harm. It is, however, an unacceptable *public* behaviour and may, therefore, be a source of difficulty and embarrassment to those around them.

If the young person already has sufficient understanding in relation to other bodily functions of the difference between those that can be carried out in public and those that cannot, the instructor will have no great problem in teaching what sexual behaviour is appropriate in public and what is not.

Excessive masturbation, so obsessive as to exclude interest in other activities, may be an indication that the daily programme of activity needs attention. Leisure activities which offer their own pleasure and satisfaction will probably reduce the need to use masturbation as the sole method of release of tension.

If the handicapped person whose masturbating is excessive is so profoundly retarded that there is no past teaching success to build upon, no possibility of using reasoned explanation or diverting energy into other activities, medical advice should be sought on possible sedation or other help. This step should be taken only where the activity is causing real distress—and this usually means distress to others. It is certainly not distressing to the masturbating individual, and to the very severely profoundly retarded person may indeed be almost the only pleasure over which he or she has personal control.

A more common problem arises from excessive displays of affection-seeking behaviour. A male staff member for instance may be troubled by a mentally handicapped young woman who follows him about and attempts to engage his attention. Sexuality after all is not expressed only in terms of biological reproductive urges, but may throughout life find outlets in other forms of creativity than procreation, in affectionate relationships with those of the opposite sex—at some stages and in some conditions to the same sex—as well as in the caring emotions of parenthood. A mentally handicapped girl may have all these elements expressed in her attempts to gain affection from a male, similarly handicapped or not. No less than her unhandicapped sisters she may make violent attachments to totally indifferent males, have maternal feelings towards babies, want to give care to another person. She may, however, not be capable of a sustained relationship. And she will not be protected against exploitation by the ability to make considered assessments of persons or circumstances. To some extent the sexuality of both young men and young women is innocent, they are reacting in a natural way to emotions they cannot understand. They have to learn, however, from attitudes of those around them, that society finds no sexual behaviour 'innocent', and has devised rules to contain the potentially destructive force inherent in sex so that the vulnerable members of the community are not at risk.

Female staff members are less concerned by excessive affection shown by mentally handicapped males—there is always more risk for male professionals, be they nurses, house-parents or teachers, in their relationships with female charges.

Female staff can usually deal with a relationship on a 'mothering' level, whereas male staff may not have a great deal of the paternal in them, and may therefore be perplexed as to how to deal with a relationship with a mentally handicapped girl who shows a sexual interest in them.

Simple caution dictates that male staff should avoid encounters where they are alone in situations which put them at risk. Before becoming too alarmed they might remember that all ordinary people are equipped to be masters of their own fate and cases of actual rape of male care staff by female patients are rare! Both male and female staff need to be aware that to be pursued by anyone involves a certain element of personal vanity, and to question whether their own behaviour may not have been open to 'misinterpretation' by a person of limited mental ability.

Sexual relationships between mentally handicapped people themselves, or with normal partners outside the caring or teaching staff, need different management.

Social and community attitudes are changing very slowly, as acceptance of mentally handicapped people in the community increases, but many long-held beliefs influence current reactions.

Some people can tolerate relationships between mentally handicapped people of any level of ability, as long as marriage is not contemplated and as long as children do not result.

Staff will find that the attitudes of parents and guardians to the awakening sexuality of their sons and daughters will vary enormously. Personal attitudes are formed by the success or failure of one's own sexual relationships, and parents and helpers may react emotionally if they are not aware of their own attitudes.

Mentally handicapped young adults will need patient individual counselling, within the ordinary social training programme. It will be necessary to include some simple explanation of the biological aspects of sexual development, of the personality changes in adolescence and the reason for the feelings of depression and euphoria—the 'highs' and 'lows' we all experience at this time in our lives.

It will be helpful if parents and helpers can demonstrate by practical example how a young man should behave if he takes a girl out on a date by helping him to choose suitable clothing, making a special effort with his toilet, washing, shaving and so on, and showing him how to walk beside a girl, offer an arm, pay for fares when travelling and at places of entertainment.

If he has always lived at home and enjoyed social outings he will have already absorbed much of this information, but whereas ordinary young people adjust their behaviour by instinctively imitating the 'courting' patterns of their peers, be they never so odd to the older generation!—the mentally handicaped young people are once again limited by their difficulty in transferring learned behaviour from one situation to another.

A whole new programme of learning has to be taught, and can only be successfully accomplished by repetition and example, and this is the task of those who are to guide the mentally handicapped boy or girl through the years from childhood into adult life.

Adolescence and young adult life is essentially a testing and proving ground for the future. Mentally handicapped young people have very much to learn before they are adult and the areas in which they need most help are those of accepted social behaviour.

LIFE SKILLS

Mentally handicapped young adults will be moving out into a complex world, fraught with many hazards in addition to the sexual ones.

Most young people, for instance, will not be able to drive a vehicle on public roads, if only because of their inability to master the Highway Code and other requirements of the driving test, though they may well achieve the needed mechanical skill to drive a tractor or a farm vehicle. So if they are not to be permanently confined by the limits of walking distance, they will need to learn to use public transport.

To quote the author of *A Long Way to Manhood* once again, Alice Candy describes in great detail the many stages of teaching her son to travel independently—and the heart-stopping anxiety she experienced before he was able to manage a journey alone. It will be necessary to make the simplest journey, a short bus ride for example, into a fully structured teaching and learning experience, especially if the young person has been in residential schools, or always been taken to school by bus or car, and has therefore very little experience of public transport. This means breaking the process down into the simplest possible steps: identifying the bus stop, then the bus; signalling the bus, boarding it and offering the right fare, etc.

Incidentally it is important not to confuse 'teaching' with 'learning'—the one does not automatically follow the other. We may think that we have taught a young adult to identify the right bus into town by showing him the number on the front of the bus. What he may be *learning* is to recognise the driver, or the advertisement on the body of the bus. General confusion arises when the driver is changed or another recognition symbol is different. Such a failure of the system gives the instructor cause to re-think his teaching method.

Money and its use may have been part of school lessons, and the young person may have learned already that goods can be bought with money, and how to calculate cost and estimate change correctly. The added skill of budgeting for essentials and making allowances for unexpected expenses may be beyond him or her. Care staff and helpers need to judge carefully how much support in these areas is needed. Groups of young adults can share skills, the more numerate doing the shopping for several others.

Eating a meal in a cafe or restaurant, with unfamiliar equipment, will also need to be taught, and appropriate behaviour when out in a group.

Young adults who have some reading and writing ability must have the opportunity to practise these skills after school is over at 16 years, and care still will need to provide time for this, and not rely upon the ubiquitous television to provide the only home activity.

Preparing a simple meal is an essential life skill, and school lessons may have included the preparation of a hot drink or toast, or other dishes. Care staff need to see that opportunities for increasing these skills are provided, and to supervise only sufficiently to ensure safety. Intelligent planning of kitchens should make it possible for handicapped people to cater for themselves to the extent to which they are able.

Personal hygiene has also usually been established by the time the young person leaves school : only the profoundly and doubly handicapped will need this service provided for them.

Menstruation and contraception techniques will need individual attention. Many mentally handicapped young women become acutely disturbed by the onset of menstruation, due to hormonal imbalance. They may have exaggerated pre-menstrual tension, especially if they are already on regular drug therapy, and this will need medical help. Behaviour disturbance may be very severe, and a girl who has previously presented problems may deteriorate temporarily into behaviour that cannot be contained in a unit with others. Good management and expert help will be needed to support her through adolescence, for public reaction to such behaviour as tearing off sanitary protection or smearing, is very strong. In the past hysterectomy was performed on women who found menstruation an impossible physical problem, but today drugs are available as an alternative.

Public expressions of affection, kissing and fondling, are on the other hand now commonly accepted among ordinary people. But mentally handicapped people, so newly accepted and warily observed by the community, are subject to more rigorous examination, and care staff need to make sure accordingly that their public behaviour is extra careful—that they understand that there is accepted public and private behaviour, even in greeting people.

They need to be shown how to dress appropriately for the occasion and how to vary their behaviour to circumstances—and they need to be given sufficient protection against exploitation, not only of a sexual character and to live with the minimum support that their abilities require.

SPECIAL DISABILITIES

As the child leaves the structured environment of school, any physical disability will become more limiting. Partial blindness, deafness and non-communicating disablement may well dictate whether or not he can live in the community or remain in institutional care. But no matter how disabling his physical condition, he will still need to be guided through the stormy waters of adolescence.

His needs for special programmes related to his physical disability must thus take into account his social and sexual needs. How this is done will depend on the degree of incapacity, and the techniques which have been employed in his school years to remedy his deficits. Care staff need to be aware of the need of the continuing evaluation of aids, and to make sure that they continue to be efficient during the period of rapid growth.

Communication is so important that care staff need to be fully familiar with alternative language systems for the non-verbal child. If such a child has been accustomed to communicate with others by means of a signing or symbol language, and is moved to an environment where no one understands him, his distress and frustration will be profoundly increased. So all institutions to which very handicapped young people come when they leave school, will need the services of a speech therapist with knowledge of alternative systems and the ability to teach them to care staff.

LEISURE

The recreation supplied by leisure activities, is an essential to mentally handicapped people as to others. Like others they will choose their leisure occupation for themselves, for the pleasure they get from them, though some will need the support of others both in the choice of activity and the way in which it is carried out.

In adolescence many new experiences are open to them. If they are physically able and have good co-ordination, they can join clubs for ordinary young people for sports such as riding, sailing and football. Their reduced ability will soon be appreciated, and in many cases they will receive friendly help from other club members to improve their performance and skill.

Riding offers a new dimension to mentally handicapped people, particularly those with allied physical handicaps. The sensation of being above the level of vision of others, and the sense of mastery of a powerful animal, may be the first opportunity that a mentally handicapped person has had of that splendid feeling of temporary superiority; and the confidence thus engendered, transfers to the rest of his regular activities.

All water sports are enjoyed, and for the young adult who has learned to swim others are immediately possible. Canoeing, sailing and water team games all provide the experience of another dimension and add to the enrichment of life.

Those who prefer less demanding physical activity may prefer to walk around their own neighbourhood, having a cup of coffee or a drink with others. Clubs for pottery, painting and other art and craft programmes may welcome a mentally handicapped member, and some Colleges of Further Education have leisure classes in cookery—for both men and women—flower arrangement, carpentry and many other activities which mentally handicapped people can join.

The Federation of Gateway Clubs nationally supervises a network of clubs specially created for mentally handicapped people, with a weekly programme of varied activities: music, dancing, a coffee bar, drama and movement classes, painting and model making, games both indoor and outdoor, excursions and in short all the activities found in clubs for ordinary young people.

Like other young adults, mentally handicapped people arriving in a new situation may be shy and unwilling to participate in an entirely new group.

Care staff should not force the issue by simply throwing the individual into unknown waters and letting him sink or swim. They should introduce him, as they would any ordinary person, to someone who is already a member of the club or group, and wait for them to become acquainted before visiting the club. It is helpful, especially in the case of a non-communicating person, to make some preliminary estimate of his abilities and preferences, so that he can be offered an activity with some immediate appeal.

Organising leisure for those who can go outside the residence is comparatively simple. Organising leisure for the profoundly handicapped person is much more difficult, but none the less essential. No one can really be said to be living if their only activities are those essential to survival. If he lies day after day in a bed, or is immobilised in a wheelchair because of his profound disability, he needs some recreation more than most. He may also need to escape from the recreation of others—continuous television or over-loud music.

For these profoundly handicapped people, nursing staff must ensure that they experience as many changes of environment as humanly possible, that they are taken out of doors at least for part of the day and allowed to feel the sun on their faces and limbs, to observe the movements of clouds and trees and leaves in the wind and see the activity of other people : gardeners, pedestrians and traffic.

Some effort should be made to find out what other activities can give them pleasure—watching mobiles (the kind designed to add interest to interior design rather than those for young children); listening to bird song or wind-moved chimes; hearing particular radio programmes; receiving a visit from an outside person who will talk to them quietly, even if they cannot respond with conversation.

If profoundly handicapped people can get around in wheelchairs, they can enjoy many other activities. Since every additional stimulation, and every widening of their experience, will increase their chance of progress, it is very important to encourage this.

Some planned physical education programmes involve the use of team skills, and some club groups have actually achieved the discipline needed to put on a display for public performance.

SECTION ELEVEN

Adult Life

Employment

Training Centres

Sheltered Employment

Open Employment

Work Preparation

Housing

Marriage

Legal Aspects

Sexual Satisfaction

Pre-marriage Counselling

Birth Control

Later Life

Senility

Death

Conclusion

Adult Life

As the young person emerges from adolescence into adult life, his needs will change. If he has received appropriate education and training he will now have achieved as a young adult, the maximum degree of independence of which he is capable. He may live in a hostel, group home, or private house in the community, he may be a resident in a village community or he may, if he is very handicapped, be living in hospital.

Wherever he lives he is now an adult, and many of the attitudes appropriate to him as a child or as an adolescent will no longer serve. To achieve the maximum degree of independence and dignity, he must be given the opportunity to choose his life style for himself; where he wishes to live, which companions he chooses, how he spends his leisure and, in some cases, his working hours.

EMPLOYMENT

There is some authoritative evidence that meaningful work is a prerequisite of full bodily and mental health for everyone. Non-handicapped adults deprived of work which contributes to the community may suffer considerable mental and emotional stress, but they may be able to adjust to the situation by creating activities for themselves. Mentally handicapped people do not have this self-starting facility, so in a sense their need for regular employment is greater.

In a time of high unemployment the less able are the least likely to find work, but the increasingly complex technology of daily life and the heightened expectations of most people today do leave some areas where opportunities of employment for mentally handicapped people can be explored. There are openings in rural crafts, in horticulture and agriculture, and in some industrial processes requiring patience rather than skill.

TRAINING CENTRES

After the Education Act of 1970 all the old Junior Training Centres for mentally handicapped children administered by Health Authorities were replaced by Special Schools, or classes.

However, the Adult Training Centre, catering for 16-year-olds upwards, continues, though some sharp enquiry into the current function of these centres is now under way. The fact remains that when the child leaves the education system at 16 or older there are few alternatives available. Opportunities for open employment, even after vocational training are hard to find, especially in times of high unemployment.

Some parents, therefore, keep young adults at home, employing them in as much household and garden activity as they can manage. Without guidance, parents do not know how to continue to develop the skills laboriously learned at school, and do not always understand that it may be necessary to reinforce reading and numeracy skills, for example, or to teach the handicapped young adult how to survive without their help—by using public transport alone or cooking simple meals for himself.

Sometimes, on the other hand, parents with high expectations will transfer them to the child, and if these are unrealistic, frustration and distress will result to both.

So home life is not always the best learning environment for the young adult who needs to discover for himself his own inner personality and to come to terms with the compromise between what he wishes, and what is possible. Some life outside the home is important for all young adults.

Young adults may attend Training Centres, now administered by the Social Services. They are staffed with managers, instructors and care staff. Many are now in a process of change from the old industrially-based concept of training to one which includes continuation of general education, self-awareness and self-expression.

Contract work was the backbone of the old ATC and managers were often rated on the success of contracts obtained and held and the subsequent revenues to the Centre. This concept is hard to

reconcile with an educational aim. In a time of high unemployment, particularly, managers have to compete for work from local
firms and must often accept work which has only a minimal
benefit to the trainee.

Trainees at an Adult Centre are not paid wages calculated upon
the amount or quality of their work, but a small sum of pocket
money set by the State—in 1979, £4 per week.

The principle behind this is that people receiving statutory
provisions—accommodation and meals—on a long-term basis,
including all residential hospital patients, can only receive a percentage of other benefits. All long-term patients, chronically sick,
aged or mentally handicapped, are deemed to have most of their
needs provided and therefore surrender other financial support
back to the State.

If the purpose of the training centre is truly for training, it needs
now to be clearly defined as training for what? There is not very
much chance of open employment for most; even work-experience
schemes, where the trainees spend some time in local industrial
units or retail outlets, do not often result in continued employment, and at times of economic recession it would be unrealistic
to expect that they should. They can have value in terms of learned social skills. Trainees can learn to work as a team, get on with
others, accept correction, travel, eat in a works canteen. This is
an educational process.

Some of the manual skills employed in contract work, too, are
useful hand-eye co-ordinating exercises, and if mastered can be
used progressively to teach sequencing programmes, essential to
such abilities as simple reading and numeracy.

The maintenance of skills already learned can also be a function of the training centre, and their development. Such work
needs a teacher seconded from the education service, or a special
class of day release at a nearby College of Further Education.
Craft instructors have been trained to impart craft skills and some
mentally handicapped people quickly master a manual skill.

The ordinary man who works at monotonous work has nevertheless mental resources of imagination which help him to use his
leisure and to plan advances and improvements to his craft tech-

niques, but mentally handicapped people do not have this same degree of independent thought, and may be stuck for years in some routine task, which may nevertheless provide for them real satisfaction.

Where there is some regular medical or nursing support at the training centre, the basic physical needs of the trainees need not devolve entirely upon the family doctor. Nursing staff can check defects of sight or hearing developing in early adult life which may be capable of correction; see that physiotherapy commenced on a regular basis in school is not totally lost in the training centre situation when its continuance is important to maintain full mobility; and see that wheelchair life is not accepted without questioning the possibility of increased mobility. They can also check on dental care and chiropody, but these services are still rare in Adult Training Centres.

The Training Centre needs new and clearly defined objectives, which can only be those of continuing education commenced at school by creating learning opportunities out of all the activities available. In-service training for staff, a new look at long-established routines, and a forward looking policy is essential.

Though designated 'training centres' they do not in fact produce 'trained' people. Only a very few enter open employment or a sheltered workshop, the very great majority will remain there for life. Nor is there planned provision for a retirement age from Adult Training Centres; ageing people return to institutional care, often to hospital.

The real problem facing the training centres is that they must perforce admit everyone regardless of levels of ability, yet they have neither funds, staff nor resources to give individual programmes to the trainees. They are neither employment centres nor educational establishments, and certainly not therapeutic centres though they need to be all three.

Some centres may have units for the very severely handicapped attached to them, called 'Special Care Units'. Some of these provide at least a daily respite for the parents who care for these adults at home, and a change of scene and new faces for those who would not otherwise be able to share in any community life.

Mentally handicapped people are driven daily by bus to the centre which is often remote from their home, and returned home at the end of the day. For those who are in wheelchairs or have other mobility problems this may be necessary; but for others this system further segregates the handicapped from the rest of the population who get themselves to work and mingle with others as they make their daily journeys.

Some new centres are in fact located near other industrial workshops on trading estates and thus provide an environment close to others at work. Occasionally the centre may undertake some stage of the production of the enterprises around them, and so make the trainees more normally accepted as part of a work force.

SHELTERED EMPLOYMENT

For some, the Training Centre may lead to sheltered employment. This may be in a specially adapted workshop, or in an industry particularly suited to the employment of handicapped persons. Blind persons, for example, can be trained as telephonists or audio typists and are extremely efficient in these roles—keeping their jobs in open employment in competition with other sighted operators.

Mentally handicapped people who are physically fit are well suited to work with farm animals, and often have great success in rearing and caring for them. Horticulture is another field available, and some rural crafts of basket making and similar activities are valuable outlets. However, if these are carried out in units entirely manned by handicapped workers, the higher proportion of supervisory staff needed means that the industry is unlikely to compete effectively in the open market so the enterprise has to be subsidised by state funds.

OPEN EMPLOYMENT

The Pathway Scheme for Open Employment employs individual mentally handicapped workers in open industry, each supported by an established member of the work force who acts as friend and instructor. This type of scheme involves a subsidy to the employer, and a payment to the nominated worker who instructs the handicapped person.

The placement officer supervises the preparation of the trainee for a short period of intensive and individual training which involves the co-operation of a specially trained staff member, who works in liaison with the employer. At the works, a member of the existing work force, who has volunteered to be responsible for the instruction and supervision of a mentally handicapped worker, will work alongside the new entrant. Close contact is maintained between the employer, placement staff member and the worker responsible for the mentally handicapped person. The success of these placements is no longer in doubt, so we can expect an extension of the system once it becomes more widely known, and more employers are willing to identify the type of work they feel can be carried out by a mentally handicapped person.

WORK PREPARATION

Our education system for the mentally handicapped is not yet properly adapted to identify the special aptitudes of an individual for certain kinds of work, and to develop these. One aim of education is to enable him to acquire the satisfaction of employment. In Sweden a highly organised system, described by Berit and Gosta Nordfors in *The Mentally Handicapped—towards normal living*, provides for identification of skills, vocational training and suitable employment. In the USSR, all citizens, including the mentally handicapped, are entitled to work when they reach school-leaving age, and special conditions are applied to the handicapped to enable them to be employed alongside other workers.

The 'right to work' is not so often invoked as the right to withdraw labour, but work is not only a right but a definite human need, and this applies to mentally handicapped people no less than to others. They must not be left out of the reckoning when the whole problem of diminishing employment prospects is under consideration and future policies discussed.

HOUSING

Happily, local authorities are making increasing provision for different types of residence within the community for those mentally handicapped adults who have been prepared for independent living.

Those living on their own for the first time need a great deal of help in understanding the need to budget for rent, rates and other essential services. Helpers also should take time to make sure that new residents have the competence to use common amenities One mentally handicapped man was constantly in need of socks, to the puzzlement of his social worker. Investigation showed that though he was quite able to use the local launderette, he had not thought of searching the drum for odd socks—and subsequent users were reaping a regular harvest of footwear! Changes in the model of cooker or refrigerator will also cause confusion, and indeed the *general* principle of 'how things work' in the home may never be understood: only how a *particular* appliance is used. Social workers and care staff need to be alert to this difficulty in transference of learning from one area to another.

Mixed sex housing units are also being provided in some areas. These tend to find themselves under particularly critical scrutiny by local citizens who would tolerate 'communes' of trendy 'normals' without comment. So care staff will need to be vigilant of standards of public social behaviour, and to encourage and support the residents for some considerable time.

For residents in community homes, privacy, a room of one's own or shared with a chosen companion is essential, as is the facility to have individual possessions and clothing secure from others. Unfortunately, there is a great variation in size of residential units, some being so large as to defy description as a 'home' in any accepted sense of the word.

Care staff should also introduce residents to local amenities— clubs, libraries, shops. Experience shows that they are usually welcomed and accepted as part of the community.

Adults who have not been used to visiting the local 'pub' and wish to do so, should be accompanied on an initial visit by a member of staff, who can explain the need for a personal drinking limit, and the custom of 'treating'. Sympathetic landlords will keep a weather eye on a new customer, and are very familiar with signs that someone has had rather more than enough, or is in unsuitable company.

It is better that residents are prepared for whatever hazards exist in their environment, than be totally sheltered from them or prohibited from participation.

Increasingly it is being understood that independence gives a positive benefit to the development of the mentally handicapped person of either sex. He is proud that he can live like others and take care of himself. His confidence increases and he becomes more independent as a result. He may even be less dependent upon community resources than the deviant 'normal', because he tends to adhere more patiently to the pattern which has been designed for him.

MARRIAGE AND MENTAL HANDICAP

People who suffer a severe disability have an added hazard in marriage, but they are not denied the right of other citizens to contract such a bond.

Legal aspects
In Britain the Registrar of marriages is required to ensure that both persons are of marriageable age or have the permission of their parents or guardians, that there is no impediment to the contract such as previous marriage, and that both parties fully understand the nature of the contract they are making. If any of these conditions is infringed the marriage may not be valid.

There is one remaining obstacle to affect the legal status of mentally handicapped people : it is still an offence under the 1956 Sexual Offenders Act to have sexual intercourse with a severely subnormal person. This stipulation is based on the assumption that a severely subnormal person is incapable of enough understanding to give valid consent either to intercourse or to the marriage contract.

It is a sufficient defence in law for an offender against the Act to say that he was not aware of the fact that his partner was severely subnormal—as we have already shown it is possible for a person who is in fact severely mentally handicapped not to appear so.

To ensure that there can be no subsequent plea by the partner of a mentally handicapped person who wishes to declare the marriage null, it is well for a mentally handicapped person to have a certificate from his doctor stating that he or she is capable of understanding the meaning of the marriage contract. Not all registrars will ask for it.

Sexual satisfaction

Among hospital residents, marriage, though still rare, is becoming more common. Those responsible for care of mentally handicapped people are aware that mutual support may improve the quality of their lives, and that sexual performance may be less important than a loving and caring relationship.

Where one partner feels that there is not sufficient sexual satisfaction, he or she may seek advice. In general, this is an area where onlookers tend to be more concerned about conformity than those actively involved. Sexual satisfaction is often related to expectation, and mentally handicapped people are less open to exhortations from the media, or to fashions in human relationships, than the rest of us. Also, in many cases, the secondary sexual emotions of loving and caring are particularly strong in partnerships of mentally handicapped people.

Pre-marriage counselling

Mentally handicapped people who are preparing to marry or to live together as common-law partners need patient counselling before setting up life together, to explain the concessions that each will have to make to the other's needs.

The personalities of both partners need to be well understood by the adviser, for each will have strengths which can be exploited for their mutual benefit, and weaknesses which will need support. There are good accounts of acceptance of the dominant role by husband or wife in the marriage situation by Michael and Ann Craft in their accounts of a number of marriages.

Sometimes the husband may be the better cook and housekeeper and the wife possess elementary skills of reading and numeracy, sometimes social work support may have to supply help in some directions until they become able to cope. There are good guidelines for those who need to undertake this work in the literature. Some sources are given in the resources appendix.

Marriage is a sufficiently hazardous undertaking for ordinary members of society—the breakdown figures, rising each year, show how many people fail to achieve success in this intimate personal relationship. Mentally handicapped people have an additional burden; but they also often have the gift of acceptance of a situation without imposed expectations. With support, many of these couples function perfectly well, helping each other to deal with the complexities of living and giving to each other the companionship and comfort expected by ordinary people who engage in a life-long contract.

Many marriages have now been studied among the mentally handicapped population and the consensus is that, with adequate support, such marriages are not only successful in themselves, but no more a charge upon community resources than marriages between 'normals'—in many cases, much less.

Birth control

Like other people, mentally handicapped adults may wish to be protected from unwanted pregnancy. If it is felt that some young women may need special protection because of their inability to understand the consequences of intercourse, a method of control must be chosen for them.

Where contraceptive advice is needed, the same options are open as to other members of society, ranging from the pill, if the wife is able to accept responsibility for this, to sterilisation by vasectomy or by ligation of the fallopian tubes, as chosen by hundreds of ordinary people.

As a general rule, it is advised that mentally handicapped people should not have children. This is not because of the risk of further increase of the handicapped population : the biological law of return to the mean—except in the case of hereditary genetic or chromosomal conditions—dictates that the children of the handicapped will tend to be closer in intelligence to the average than their parents; but because of the reduced ability of the parents particularly the mother, to cope with the demands of the infant and child.

All oestrogen based contraceptives have some side effects, and it is necessary for medical advice to give the original prescription and also to monitor the side effects.

A mechanical device inserted into the womb (IUD) may be preferred, but again this needs to be monitored by medical staff to ensure that it is effective and is not causing injury.

Any female requiring contraceptive advice should be regularly advised, and the method selected according to her ability to understand what is required.

Males may be instructed to use a mechanical barrier, a sheath, but this requires considerable instruction and is not practicable in most cases. Where a wife cannot be protected, vasectomy is the most likely method to be advised for the male partner.

DEVIANT SEXUAL BEHAVIOUR

Some mentally handicapped men, in common with some other men, find satisfaction in indecent exposure. A prosecution for this offence is based on the premise that it causes disgust and annoyance, whether or not there was intent to cause it. It is on these grounds that men are prosecuted for urinating in public. There is no need to prove intent to offend to secure a conviction.

In the case of the mentally handicapped male, it would be self-apparent that his action was not specifically designed to cause disgust or annoyance, but the only defence would be that he was not responsible for his own actions. If he were to use this defence, however, he might find himself the subject of an order for confinement in a place of safety, rather than the fine which would be the penalty for ordinary people. So it is clearly the duty of those in care of mentally handicapped people who are not able to understand socially acceptable behaviour to protect them from such charges by any available means.

There is still some confusion about the position of staff with respect to sexual relations with residents of either sex whilst they are in a patient/therapist relationship; and the confusion is worse confounded by the various legal ages of consent, for heterosexual relationships on the one hand and consenting adult males in a homosexual relationship on the other.

In general, staff are well advised to regard all residents in their care as in a special relationship. Whilst providing every opportunity for social intercourse between residents and the outside community, they should always be aware that society will watch every tentative foray into the field of 'normalisation' and nowhere will criticism be so sharp in the area of sexual relationships. Professional ethics for all care staff should be sufficiently clear and carefully observed to protect both residents and staff.

LATER LIFE

A particular problem is that of the mentally handicapped person in the community who has always lived at home, then on the death of one parent, or both, is left without home or support. It is usually the mother who has cared for the handicapped person, so a father left alone simply cannot manage. In other cases, particularly if the handicapped person is heavy, disturbed or otherwise difficult, the death of the father is the final blow and the mother cannot cope alone.

Social Services need to be aware of mentally handicapped people living with ageing parents, and to anticipate the situation which may arise when the parents are no longer able to cope. Short-term stay away from home in the type of amenity which will probably be most suitable is a useful preparation, and may spare much anxiety later.

These people can be of very different levels of ability. If there is profound retardation or very severe physical impairment, there may be no alternative to hospital care. But mentally handicapped people removed to hospital after many years at home have a great deal of distress and personal misery to overcome, no matter how kindly the arrangement is made. So wherever possible, family visitors should be encouraged to make regular and frequent visits, so that hospital staff can discuss points of difficulty. For instance, changes in routine can cause quite violent behaviour changes and it may be possible to minimise these if the home routine is known.

The ability to adapt to change becomes less as age advances, and it is especially necessary to make a transition as gradually as possible if the handicapped person is no longer young.

Less severely handicapped people may be able to live in hostels or group homes in their own town, where their knowledge of local shops and transport will be an asset to them.

Senility

In common with the rest of the population, mentally handicapped people will require care in old age. At this stage of their lives, their condition will approximate closely to that of other aged persons requiring special care. Premature ageing, however, is a feature of some conditions and relatively young people, in their late fifties, will already exhibit the symptoms of advanced age and will need extra care.

So far, no authority has planned any special provision for aged mentally handicapped persons. They are still expected to re-enter the subnormality hospital rather than the geriatric wards of general hospitals, but this again is something which may change in the future. Their needs will be identical with others at this stage.

Death

People are apt to think that, because they have difficulty in expressing emotions and thoughts, mentally handicapped people are incapable of appreciating the fact of death or of feeling the loss of someone close to them, relative or neighbour, or friend in a ward or hostel.

In fact it is well established that the mentally handicapped do indeed experience sorrow and grief, even if it is often expressed not in words but by marked personality and behaviour changes. Their capacity to understand and rationalise such an event is

G

reduced, but care staff need to understand the need for comfort, explanation and reassurance, and for an outlet for grief. It is more difficult for the mentally handicapped than for others to share sorrow—the initiative to do so must come from those who care for them.

CONCLUSION

So much has been introduced in this brief guide, that it is certain that more questions have been provoked than answers provided.

In short, the changing needs of mentally handicapped people and the new techniques available to help them require imagination from all the caring staff and those who plan and administer the many community services.

Fortunately many others have gathered specialised knowledge of mental handicap, and of techniques and practices applicable to the variety of problems which the condition presents.

The list of books and resources which follows will expand the sections most applicable to the particular needs of the student. This small book sets the door ajar—it will open wider and wider, revealing new horizons for those who care enough to explore further the fascinating world of the mentally handicapped.

Bibliography and Resource Material

In these lists will be found reference material at every level, from brief pamphlets on particular topics, to standard texts for students and consultants.

It is not possible to indicate which book will best serve a particular need but students may find some general advice helpful.

No book can solve a problem. It may help to define the true nature of the problem and indicate possible solutions, so unless you know what you want to discover, you may waste time searching endless text books.

Faced with, for example, six medical text books written for varying levels of comprehension, it may help if you select one topic, say 'mongolism' from the index, and read the entry under this topic, in each. You will at least find which writer makes the answer most clear to you and that, therefore, it is likely that that particular book will be the one you can use. When seeking a quick answer or reference, look first in any good general dictionary or encyclopaedia for a concise explanation. Words in general use, genes, chromosomes, diphtheria, syndrome, retardation, psychology and other common terms are quickly defined in this way and the short definition will often lead the student to the further information he may need.

Remember that the Librarian in your training school, or public library, has access to a vast store of knowledge, and can help to trace any published material. If you know which book you want, you can request that it be obtained for you by any public library, but make sure that all the vital information, Author, Title, Publisher and year of publication is given on your request, and be prepared to wait for a little for the book to arrive at your library.

In addition to the books listed, many organisations publish

pamphlets giving concise information and suggestions for practical help to parents. Relevant addresses are given in the Resource Section.

The National Society for Mentally Handicapped Children has a comprehensive list of these, including topics such as phenyl-ketonuria, speech therapy, mongolism, helping children to under-stand sexuality, to learn at home and infant management. A complete list is available.

The Health Education Council produces leaflets and booklets, many of which are free. Some useful new titles are 'Weaning', 'Can't Talk Yet', 'Care of Young Feet'. Current titles are listed, and the list can be obtained from the Council free of charge.

The Down's Children's Association has a list of very helpful publications for parents.

The Disabled Living Foundation have excellent information sheets on wheelchair aids, special clothing and many other aspects of daily care for those with physical handicap.

GENERAL INFORMATION on all aspects of mental handicap can be obtained from the Information Officer, NSMHC, 117, Golden Lane, London. EC1Y 0RT. Tel : 01-253 9433.

Bibliography

OFFICE OF HEALTH ECONOMICS. (1973). *Mental Handicap*. Office of Health Economics, 162 Regent Street, London W1R 6DD.

H.M.S.O. *Better Services for the Mentally Handicapped*. (1971).

DEPARTMENT OF HEALTH AND SOCIAL SECURITY. *Helping Mentally Handicapped People in Hospital*. (1978).

H.M.S.O. *Report of the Jay Committee into Mental Handicap Nursing and Care*. (1979).

Developmental progress

GESSELL, A. (1950). *The First Five Years of Life. A Guide to the Study of the Pre-School Child*. Methuen.

GESSELL, A. & Catherine S. Amatruda. (1941/1947). *Developmental Diagnosis. Normal and Abnormal Child Development— Clinical Methods and Pediatric Applications*. Harper & Row.

SHERIDAN, Mary D. (1975). *Children's Developmental Progress from Birth to Five Years: the Stycar Sequences*. NFER Publishing Co. Ltd.

Children at home

COLLINS, M. & Doreen. (1976). *Kith and Kids—self-help for families of the handicapped*. Souvenir Press.

CROZIER, M. *Stress in families with mentally handicapped children*. NSMHC.

CUNNINGHAM, C. & Patricia Sloper. (1978). *Helping Your Handicapped Child*. Souvenir Press.

SHERIDAN, Mary D. (1975). *The Handicapped Child and his Home*. National Children's Home.

Pamphlets

The Specialised Health Visitor for the Handicapped Baby, Young Child and School Child. Report published by the Disabled Living Foundation. (1979).

You and Your Baby. British Medical Association Handbooks.

Make the Most of Your Baby. Mather, J. (1976). NSMHC.

Lesley, The Child We Chose. Smithson, M. (1977). NSMHC.
Help Your Child to Learn at Home. Shennan, V. (1978). NSMHC.
Helping the Handicapped Child in the Family. Jobling, M. NFER.
Towards Normal Skills. Michaelis, G. (1978). NSMHC.

Education

LORTON, J. W. & B. L. Walley. (1979). *Introduction to Early Childhood Education*. D. Van Nostrand Co., New York.
BROOKS, Barbara. *Teaching Mentally Handicapped Children*. Ward Lock Educational.
CUMMINGS, P. (1973). *Education and the Severely Handicapped Child*. NSMHC.
BALL, F. (1978). *The Development of Reading Skills*. Blackwell.
NORRIS, D. (1975). *Day Care and Severe Handicap*. NSMHC.

Speech and language development

AINLEY, J., B. Atteridge, C. Catchpole & R. Clarke. (1978). *Early Language Programme*. Royal Borough of Kingston-upon-Thames.
DEICH, R. F. & P. M. Hodges. (1977). *Language without Speech*. Souvenir Press.
GILLHAM, B. (1979). *The First Words Language Programme*. Allen & Unwin and Beaconsfield Publishers.
JEFFREE, Dorothy & R. McConkey. (1977). *Let Me Speak*. Souvenir Press.
LURIA, A. R. & F. La Yudovitch. (1975). *Penguin Papers in Education*. Penguin Education.
SHENNAN, Victoria (1978). *Russian Education for the Retarded* NSMHC.

Pamphlet
Language Stimulus with Retarded Children. La Frenais, M. (1971). NSMHC.

Play

JEFFREE, Dorothy, R. McConkey & S. Hewson. (1977). *Let Me Play*. Souvenir Press.
PLANNED PARENTHOOD ASSOCIATION. *Guidelines for Playgroups with a Handicapped Child*. (1978).
SHERIDAN, Mary D. (1977). *Spontaneous Play in Early Childhood from Birth to Six Years*. NFER Publishing Co. Ltd.

Pamphlets
Stimulation Through Play. Baum, L. (1977). NSMHC.
Making Movement Fun. Mortimore, F. (1978). NSMHC.

Hospital
CASS, H. et al. *Take Six Children.* (1978). NSMHC.
DEACON, J. J. (1974). *Tongue Tied.* NSMHC.
Required reading for all students. Autobiography of a patient describing 50 years of life in a subnormality hospital.
GIBSON, J. & T. French. (1977). *Nursing the Mentally Retarded.* Faber.
HALES, Ann. (1978). *Children of Skylark Ward.* Cambridge University Press.
KING EDWARD'S HOSPITAL FUND FOR LONDON. *Living in Hospital.*
LANCASTER MOOR HOSPITAL. *Glossary of Terms, Tests and Drugs used in Psychiatric Practice.* (1958). Administrator, Lancaster Moor Hospital, Lancaster.
MITTLER, Professor P. (1978). *Helping Mentally Handicapped People in Hospital.* Department of Health and Social Security.
HALES, Ann. (1978). *Children of Skylark Ward.* Cambridge University Press.
PAINE, L. (1972). *Know your Hospital.* British Hospital Journal in conjunction with Heinemann Medical Books.
H.M.S.O. *Report of the Health Services Commissioner, December 1978 to March 1979.* (Records submissions of malpractice by NHS staff).
H.M.S.O. Report. *The Education of Children in Hospitals for the Mentally Handicapped.* Dec., 1978.

Clinical
RICHARDS, B. W. (Ed.) (1970). *Mental Subnormality. Modern Trends in Research.* Pitman Medical & Scientific Publishing Co.
STAFFORD-CLARK, D. & A. C. Smith. (1979). *Psychiatry for Students.* Allen & Unwin.
(New edition under preparation with complete revision of the section on mental handicap.)
WING, Lorna. (1975). *Autistic Children.* Constable.
WING, Lorna. *Early Childhood Autism.* (1976). Pergamon Press.

Pamphlets
The Child with Phenylketonuria. Tyfield & Holton. (1974). NSMHC.
Down's Syndrome. L. Lowenstein. (1978). NSMHC.

Psychology
COMLEY, J. (1975). *Behaviour Modification with the Retarded Child.* Heinemann Medical Books.

ROBINSON, H. B. & M. Robinson. (1965). *The Mentally Retarded Child*. McGraw Hill.

SANDSTROM, C. I. (1979). *The Psychology of Childhood and Adolescence*. Penguin Books.

THOMAS, D. (1978). *Social Psychology of Childhood Disability*. Methuen.

WEIHS, T. J. (1978). *Children in Need of Special Care*. Souvenir Press.

KIERNAN, C., & Jones, M. (1977). *Behaviour Assessment Battery*. NFER.

Residential care

OSWIN, Maureen. (1978). *Holes in the Welfare Net*. Bedford Square Press.

SHENNAN, Victoria. (1979). (Ed.) *Directory of Residential Accommodation for the Mentally Handicapped in England, Wales and Northern Ireland*. NSMHC.

McCORMACK, Mary. (1979). *Away from Home: The Mentally Handicapped in Residential Care*. Constable.

Health

HEALTH EDUCATION COUNCIL. Current Publications List.

MURRAY, A. (1976). *Look After Yourself*. Health Education Council.

SJEET, M. & E. Crout. (1977). *Health Needs Help*. Blackwell Scientific Publications.

Safety first and first aid

British Red Cross and St. John Ambulanct Brigade Handbooks. (Apply also to local branch for training courses.)

Sport and leisure

UPTON, G. (1979). *Physical and Creative Activities for the Mentally Handicapped*. Cambridge University Press.

GROVES, L. (1979). *Physical Education for Special Needs*. Cambridge University Press.

GUTTMAN, Sir L. (1976). *Sport for the Physically Handicapped*. UNESCO, Paris.

Pamphlets

Recreation for the Retarded. (A Leader's Handbook). Stuart, F. (1975). NSMHC.

A Philosophy of Leisure in Relation to the Retarded. Solly, K. (1975). NSMHC.

Staff and training
HEGARTY, J. R., & S. P. Winter. (Eds.) (1978). *Educating the Trainers*. Conference Proceedings. Department of Psychology.
MALIN, N. *Staff Attitudes in Mental Handicap*. Scottish Society for the Mentally Handicapped.
OFFICE OF HEALTH ECONOMICS. (1973). *Mental Handicap*. Office of Health Economics, 162 Regent Street, London W1R 6DD.

Pamphlets
Sex and Social Training in an Adult Training Centre. Lowes, L. (1977). NSMHC.
Sex Education and the Mentally Retarded. Lee, G. W. (1977). NSMHC.
Help Your Child to Understand Sex. Shennan, V. (1977). NSMHC.

Adult life
BARANYAY, Eileen P. (1971). *The Mentally Handicapped Adolescent*. Pergamon Press.
BARANYAY, Eileen P. (1976). *A Lifetime of Learning*. NSMHC.
BBC. (1978). *Let's Go*—notes for parents and instructors to accompany TV series on social skills for the mentally handicapped. BBC Publications.
CRAFT, M. & Ann. (1978). *Sex and the Mentally Handicapped*. Routledge & Kegan Paul.
GRUNEWALD, K. (1978). *The Mentally Handicapped. Towards Normal Living*. Hutchinson.
GITTINS, S. G. (Ed.) (1974). *The Educational Needs of Mentally Handicapped Adults*. Report of a Joint Conference 1974. NSMHC.
HENSHAW, Anne. (1979). *After Sixteen*. NSMHC.
TUCKEY, Linda, Jessie Parfitt & B. Tuckey. (1973). *Handicapped School Leavers—their further education, training and employment*. NFER Publishing Co. Ltd.
WHELAN, E. & Barbara Speacke. (1979). *Learning to Cope*. Souvenir Press.

Pamphlet
A Long Way to Manhood. Candy, A. (1976). NSMHC.

Statutory provisions, United Kingdom
The Acts below are those which are most likely to affect mentally handicapped people.
Mental Health Act 1959.

Chronically Sick and Disabled Persons Act 1970.
Local Authority Social Services Act 1970.
Education (Handicapped Children) Act 1970.

Reports

When changing conditions require an amendment to Statutes, the Government of the day sets up a 'Royal Commission' or 'Special Committee' to consider changes in the law. These bodies then report to Government, and their findings, conclusions and recommendations are published. Subsequent changes to legislation may follow.

Reports currently available are :
Better Services for the Mentally Handicapped, 1971.
Fit for the Future (The Court Report), 1976.
Special Educational Needs (The Warnock Report), 1976.
Report of the Committee of Enquiry into Mental Handicap Nursing and Care (The Jay Report), 1979.
A Review of the Mental Health Act 1959, 1978.
Report of the Royal Commission into the N.H.S., 1979
A Service for Patients – conclusions and recommendations from the Royal Commission, 1979

Copies can be obtained from H.M. Stationery Office.

International services

Care of the Mentally Retarded in the Community. Conference Report. June 1974. Regional Office for Europe, WHO, Copenhagen. A brief account of the statutory service available at that date in France, Spain, Sweden, USSR and UK, with organisational structures of the voluntary organisations in Australia, Canada, New Zealand, UK and USA.

Organisation of Services for the Mentally Retarded. Fifteenth Report of the WHO Expert Committee on Mental Health, Geneva 1960. Technical Report No. 392. The collective views of an international group of experts from many countries including Pakistan, Japan, USSR, Belgium, Uruguay, USA and UK. Gives recommendations on many aspects including classification, nomenclature, education and training, legal aspects and public education.

The Law and Mental Health: Harmonizing Objectives. Curran, W. J., Harding, T. W. WHO Geneva 1978. A comparative survey of existing legislation, worldwide, with guidelines for assessment and alternative approaches to improving the laws affecting mentally handicapped people.

Resources

Information on the resources quoted may not always be up to date. Addresses can change very quickly, but once the correct title of the organisation or service is known, recourse to the current Directories will give the up-to-date information. Your local librarian will help you to find what you need.

If you approach a voluntary body for help remember that you will need to define your questions first, the same is true for the statutory agencies. A vague and ill-defined query shows that you have not really thought about the subject.

As you increase your practical knowledge of mental handicap, you will find that you evaluate what you read about the condition against what you have yourself learned and observed, and will perhaps have original and valuable contributions to make to the sum of knowledge.

Films
Concorde Films, Nacton, Ipswich, have a comprehensive catalogue of films for hire. There are a number on mental handicap, including a new film, 'In a World Apart', 1979, NSMHC.

HESTER ADRIAN RESEARCH CENTRE
The University of Manchester, Manchester M13 9PL
Tel: 061-273 3333

THE BRITISH INSTITUTE OF MENTAL SUBNORMALITY
Wolverhampton Road, Kidderminster. Worcs
Tel: 0562 850251

KING'S FUND CENTRE
126 Albert Street, London NW1 7NF
Tel: 01-267 6111/2

KITH & KIDS
6 Grosvenor Road, London N10
Tel: 01-883 8762

MIND (NATIONAL ASSOCIATION FOR MENTAL HEALTH)
22 Harley Street, London W1N 2ED
Tel : 01-637 0741.

NATIONAL ASSOCIATION OF TEACHERS FOR THE
MENTALLY HANDICAPPED
1 Beechfield Avenue, Urmston, Manchester
Tel : 061-748 2123

NATIONAL CHILDREN'S BUREAU
8 Wakley Street, London EC1V 7QE
Tel : 01-278 9441

NATIONAL COUNCIL FOR SPECIAL EDUCATION
1 Wood Street, Stratford-on-Avon
Tel : 78-89 5332

NATIONAL FEDERATION OF GATEWAY CLUBS
117-123 Golden Lane, London EC1Y 0RT
Tel : 01-253 9433

NATIONAL SOCIETY FOR MENTALLY HANDICAPPED
CHILDREN
117-123 Golden Lane, London EC1Y 0RT.

PRE-SCHOOL PLAYGROUPS ASSOCIATION
Alford House, Aveline Street, London SE11 5DJ
Tel : 01-582 8871

RIDING FOR THE DISABLED
Avenue 'R'
National Agriculture Centre
Kenilworth, Waks CV8 2LY.
Tel : 0203-56107

SCOTTISH SOCIETY FOR THE
MENTALLY HANDICAPPED
13 Elmbank Street, Glasgow G2 4QA, Scotland
Tel : 041-226 4541

SESAME
George Bell House
8 Ayres Street, London SE1 1ES
Tel : 01-407 2159

SPASTICS SOCIETY
12 Park Crescent, London W1
Tel : 01-636 5020

TOY LIBRARIES ASSOCIATION
Seabrook House
Willyotts Manor
Darkes Lane, Potters Bar, Herts
Tel : 77-44571

Index